PERFORMANCE-
EN
D

Other books in the At Issue series:

Alcohol Abuse
Animal Experimentation
Anorexia
The Attack on America: September 11, 2001
Biological and Chemical Weapons
Bulimia
The Central Intelligence Agency
Cloning
Creationism vs. Evolution
Does Capital Punishment Deter Crime?
Drugs and Sports
Drunk Driving
The Ethics of Abortion
The Ethics of Genetic Engineering
The Ethics of Human Cloning
Heroin
Home Schooling
How Can Gun Violence Be Reduced?
How Should Prisons Treat Inmates?
Human Embryo Experimentation
Is Global Warming a Threat?
Islamic Fundamentalism
Is Media Violence a Problem?
Legalizing Drugs
Missile Defense
National Security
Nuclear and Toxic Waste
Nuclear Security
Organ Transplants
Physician-Assisted Suicide
Police Corruption
Professional Wrestling
Rain Forests
Satanism
School Shootings
Should Abortion Rights Be Restricted?
Should There Be Limits to Free Speech?
Teen Sex
Video Games
What Encourages Gang Behavior?
What Is a Hate Crime?
White Supremacy Groups

PERFORMANCE-ENHANCING DRUGS

James Haley, *Book Editor*

Daniel Leone, *President*
Bonnie Szumski, *Publisher*
Scott Barbour, *Managing Editor*

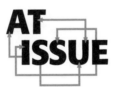

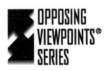

THOMSON
™
GALE

San Diego • Detroit • New York • San Francisco • Cleveland
New Haven, Conn. • Waterville, Maine • London • Munich

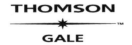

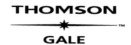

LIBRARY OF CONGRESS CATALOGING-IN-PUBLICATION DATA

Performance-enhancing drugs / James Haley, book editor.
  p. cm. — (At issue)
Includes bibliographical references and index.
ISBN 0-7377-1170-1 (lib. : alk. paper) — ISBN 0-7377-1169-8 (pbk. : alk. paper)
  1. Doping in sports. I. Title: Performance-enhancing drugs. II. Haley, James,
1968– . III. At issue (San Diego, Calif.)
RC1230 .P475 2003
362.29'088'796—dc21

          2002028600

Contents

Page

Introduction   7

1. Performance-Enhancing Drugs: An Overview   11
   Craig Freudenrich

2. Athletes Will Never Stop Using Performance-Enhancing Drugs   20
   Matt Barnard

3. Athletes Must Stop Using Performance-Enhancing Drugs   24
   Merrell Noden

4. Performance-Enhancing Drugs Tarnish Athletics   28
   European Commission

5. The Ban on Performance-Enhancing Drugs Should Continue   35
   Economist

6. Teen Steroid Abuse Is a Growing Problem   41
   Steven Ungerleider

7. Performance-Enhancing Drugs Compromise Medical Ethics   45
   Philippe Liotard

8. Performance-Enhancing Drugs Should Be Regulated, Not Prohibited   50
   Malcolm Gladwell

9. Ban Athletes Who Don't Use Steroids   60
   Sidney Gendin

10. Coming Soon: Open Olympics!   62
    Oliver Morton

11. The Health Risks of Steroid Use Have Been Exaggerated   65
    Rick Collins

12. One Strike, You're Out   76
    Mark Starr

13. Performance-Enhancing Drug Testing Is Ineffective   79
    Anonymous

14. Performance-Enhancing Dietary Supplements Are   88
    Dangerous
    Gwen Knapp

15. Performance-Enhancing Dietary Supplements Are Safe   91
    Council for Responsible Nutrition

16. Genetic Engineering May One Day Replace Performance-   94
    Enhancing Drugs
    Jere Longman

Organizations to Contact   102

Bibliography   106

Index   109

Introduction

The Tour de France is considered the world's most competitive bicycle race. Each summer top cycling teams from around the world compete in the three-week event, which sends riders on a grueling, multi-stage course through the mountainous countryside of Ireland, France, and Belgium. In 1998, the image of Tour de France cyclists as athletes at the peak of their natural abilities was tarnished by allegations of widespread performance-enhancing drug use among competitors. The "doping" scandal broke a few days prior to the start of the race when a masseuse for France's Festina team, Willy Voet, was arrested after police found large quantities of anabolic steroids and erythropoietin, or EPO, in his car as he crossed from Belgium into France. A subsequent police investigation uncovered a well-organized system, orchestrated by the team's management and doctor, for supplying riders with illicit performance-enhancing drugs. The Festina team was suspended from the Tour, and further investigations by French police led to the suspension and withdrawal of several more teams. Riders went on strike to protest the investigations, and less than half of the original competitors finished the race.

French authorities are not alone in punishing athletes who use performance-enhancing drugs. From the International Olympic Committee (IOC) to the National Basketball Association (NBA) to the National Collegiate Athletics Association (NCAA), most high-profile sports organizations have taken substantial steps to crack down on doping. Stronger anti-doping initiatives are considered necessary to preclude scandals that damage the image of sports and to silence critics who contend that not enough is being done to rid sports of drugs. The IOC, for example, which enforces the rules of the Olympic Games, set up the World Anti-Doping Agency (WADA) in 1999 as an independent body charged with coordinating a consistent system for testing Olympic athletes. WADA works with international sports federations and Olympic committees and has begun conducting unannounced, out-of-competition tests on Olympic hopefuls. This practice reduces the chance that competitors will rid their systems of drugs before being tested. The list of banned substances on the Olympic Movement's Anti-Doping Code includes stimulants, narcotics, anabolic steroids, beta blockers, diuretics, various hormones, and drugs known as "masking agents," which are used to prevent detection of illicit substances during drug tests. WADA is also investing more of its resources in developing new tests to keep pace with the changing array of drugs that athletes are taking.

Whether or not those who contend that drug tests remain easy to beat will be satisfied by renewed testing efforts remains uncertain. Clearly, however, performance-enhancing drug testing has affected the careers of many elite athletes. Athletes who test positive for drugs at the Olympic level are stripped of their medals and records and are suspended from all competition for two years on the first offense. In 1988, Canadian sprinter Ben Johnson was stripped of a gold medal and was later banned from track-and-field competition for life after he tested positive for steroids. At the 2000 Summer Olympic Games in Sydney, Australia, Romanian gymnast Andrea Raducan had her gold medal taken away when she tested positive for pseudoephedrine, a stimulant. American shot-putter C.J. Hunter withdrew from competition after it was revealed that he had tested positive four times for the steroid nandrolone. Scores of other athletes were also expelled from the Sydney Games after flunking drug tests. More recently, at the 2002 Winter Olympic Games in Salt Lake City, Utah, British skier Alain Baxter was stripped of his bronze medal after testing positive for methamphetamine, although an appeal is pending.

Detection efforts notwithstanding, seeking an edge over one's opponents has long made the use of performance-enhancing drugs a part of athletic competition. A review of sports history reveals that drugs and sports have gone hand-in-hand for centuries, and surprisingly, drugs have only been banned from the Olympic Games since 1968. Explains Ivan Waddington in his book *Sport, Health, and Drugs*, "Performance-enhancing drugs have been used by people involved in sport and sport-like activities for some 2,000 years, but it is only very recently (specifically, since the introduction of anti-doping regulations and doping controls from the 1960s) that this practice has been regarded as unacceptable. In other words, for all but the last three or four decades, those involved in sports have used performance-enhancing drugs without infringing any rules and without the practice giving rise to highly emotive condemnation and stigmatization." This shift from tolerating doping in sports to testing athletes and ostracizing drug cheats has been driven by several factors. Perhaps most important, technological advances in performance-enhancing drugs, beginning in the 1950s, have bolstered the contention that drug use threatens the integrity of sports. Another motivation behind the shift has been to deter athletes from using illicit substances with unknown health effects.

Consider, for example, the evolution of performance-enhancing drugs. Athletes in the late-nineteenth and early-twentieth centuries looking for chemical enhancement were stuck with the limited efficacy of stimulants and painkillers. In the mid-1950s, anabolic steroids, synthetic versions of the male sex hormone testosterone, were introduced. Anabolic steroids build muscle and bone mass by stimulating the muscle and bone cells to make new protein. Coaches and athletes saw these drugs as a major breakthrough because they enabled athletes to transcend the limits of natural ability and reach new levels of competitiveness.

The first indication that athletes were using steroids came during the 1956 World Games in Moscow, Russia. According to Robert Voy in his book *Drugs, Sport, and Politics*, an American doctor, John B. Ziegler, observed Soviet athletes using urinary catheters, because steroids had enlarged their prostates to the point where urination was difficult. Ziegler returned to the United States and helped develop Dianobol, a steroid that was quickly embraced by American athletes, who hoped it would level the playing field with the Soviets. As a result, steroid use became widespread among elite athletes.

Concerns that doped athletes were exercising an unfair advantage over their opponents and violating the ideals of sportsmanship followed the rise in steroid use. Explains John Hoberman, the author of *Mortal Engines: The Science of Performance and the Dehumanization of Sport,* "Performance-enhancing drugs have subverted this ideal [of sportsmanship] in two distinct ways. First, many athletes have abandoned self-restraint in this regard, resulting in a crisis of *conduct,* such as Ben Johnson's disgrace as a 'cheater.' Second, the scientization of the athlete, either through drugs or other techniques, also involves a crisis of *identity.* . . . To what extent can the emotional experience of competition be truly shared with an athlete who has transformed himself . . . with drugs? . . . Once the athlete has abandoned self-restraint, drug testing becomes the sole guarantor of the 'integrity' of sport." Sports authorities and fans came to understand that technology would inevitably provide athletes with an endless array of pharmaceutical enhancements. Controls had to be placed on doping in order to prevent sports from becoming a science laboratory where the human spirit played second fiddle to pills and injections. It is also important to keep in mind that as of 1990, following federal legislation, the use of anabolic steroids became illegal without a prescription, and possession can bring heavy fines and prison terms for users and dealers. Breaking the law to stay competitive is regarded by many observers as a further affront to the ideals of sportsmanship.

In addition to upholding the integrity of sports by expunging cheaters, drug testing is done to deter athletes from participating in a "race to the bottom" as far as their health is concerned. If performance-enhancing drugs were permitted in all sports competitions, contend supporters of the drug ban, athletes would have to become virtual guinea pigs in order to remain competitive. And because athletes regularly take larger doses of steroids and other drugs than medical patients, the long-term health effects of such drug use are unknown. Health reports from some athletes exposed to performance-enhancing drugs offer reason for caution. Greg Strock, a member of the U.S. Olympic cycling team in the early 1990s, alleges that coaches, without his consent, doped him with steroid injections. Strock attributes the breakdown of his immune system and the end of his promising cycling career to large doses of the drugs. Christiane Knacke-Sommer, a swimmer with the East German Olympic team in the 1970s, was given regular injections of testosterone, a male hormone, without her knowledge. In 1998, she testified in a trial against her former coaches that the treatments "destroyed my body and my mind," and permanently masculinized her physique and voice.

However, many athletes are willing to chance these health risks, and they take issue with assertions that there is something unfair or unnatural about using performance-enhancing drugs. They argue that drug use is one advantage among many, such as access to superior coaching or training facilities, that athletes may or may not have at their disposal to sharpen their competitive edge. The fact that all athletes are not starting with the same set of advantages discredits the notion that a "level playing field" can somehow be restored if drugs are eliminated. According to this view, performance-enhancing drugs are simply making up for an athlete's natural deficiencies or quality of training.

Another argument put forth by athletes is that elite sporting events are so demanding that competing in them virtually necessitates drug use. Revelations that Tour de France riders were doping themselves surprised some fans of the sport, but riders who admit to drug use are more matter-of-fact. They contend that without drugs like EPO, which enhances athletic endurance by boosting the amount of oxygen in the blood, competing in the Tour de France would be nearly impossible. Nicolas Aubier, a former French professional cyclist, explains the rationale behind drug use in the book *Rough Ride: Behind the Wheel with a Pro Cyclist,* by Paul Kimmage: "To be honest, I don't think it's possible to make the top 100 on the ranking list without taking EPO, growth hormone or some of the other stuff."

The desire to remain competitive among athletes goes a long way toward explaining their willingness to use performance-enhancing drugs. At the beginning of the twenty-first century, athletic achievement is esteemed by millions of fans the world over, who eagerly watch satellite feeds of sporting events in anticipation of the next world record. Sponsors pay millions of dollars to have their products prominently advertised at sports arenas or endorsed by athletes. In this environment, as Karen Goldberg, a reporter with the magazine *Insight on the News*, asserts, athletes are under a tremendous amount of pressure to perform. Writes Goldberg, "As the stakes became higher, so did the number of athletes who sought performance-enhancing drugs, spurred on by the lure of big contracts and lucrative endorsements."

Keeping drugs out of athletic competition has only become more difficult for sports authorities since drug testing was introduced to the Olympic Games in 1968. Changing social norms and technology, which spurred the initial drive to ban drugs in sports, may end up settling the debate. Western societies have shown increasing tolerance for using drugs to enhance performance in areas of life outside of athletics. Drugs such as Viagra, Prozac, and Ritalin are now regularly prescribed to improve sexual, social, and academic performance. It may simply be a matter of time before the "integrity" of athletics no longer appears threatened by performance-enhancing drugs, particularly if safer drugs are developed. The ethical debate over whether or not athletes should use performance-enhancing drugs is one of the issues discussed in *At Issue: Performance-Enhancing Drugs*. Other issues include the effectiveness of drug testing, the rise of steroid use among teenage athletes, and the dangers of dietary supplements.

1

Performance-Enhancing Drugs: An Overview

Craig Freudenrich

Craig Freudenrich is a biomedical researcher and a senior editor of science, medicine, and the human body for the website HowStuffWorks.com.

Many athletes have turned to performance-enhancing drugs to gain a competitive advantage. Performance-enhancing drugs include anabolic steroids for building mass and strength, and protein hormones that increase the amount of oxygen in body tissues, which boosts athletic endurance. Most of these drugs have unpleasant and/or dangerous side effects and have been banned by the International Olympic Committee and other governing athletic agencies. Urine and blood tests are conducted to keep drug users out of athletic competitions, but "masking drugs" are often taken to hide the presence of illegal substances, making detection difficult.

Every two years as the Olympic Games begin, we hear about athletes using or, at least, being tested for performance-enhancing drugs. Sometimes, competitors raise the question when one athlete does particularly well. Other times, tests catch athletes with drugs in their systems. The practice of using artificial substances or methods to enhance athletic performance is called doping. Doping has become such a great concern that the United States formed the U.S. Anti-Doping Agency (USADA) in October 2000.

This viewpoint discusses why some athletes take drugs, what the major classes of drugs and their side effects are and how drug use is tested. Although there is no statistical evidence about how widespread doping is, athletes and coaches stress that most competitors do not take drugs. This viewpoint will help [people] . . . who are concerned about young athletes who might be influenced to try doping. You will learn the names and effects of the drugs as well as ways that the drugs are detected.

Why some athletes use drugs

Athletes face enormous pressure to excel in competition. They also know that winning can reap them more than a gold medal. A star athlete can earn a lot of money and a lot of fame, and athletes only have a short time to do their best work. Athletes know that training is the best path to victory, but they also get the message that some drugs and other practices can boost their efforts and give them a shortcut, even as they risk their health and their athletic careers.

As far back as ancient Greece, athletes have often been willing to take any preparation that would improve their performance. But it appears that drug use increased in the 1960s. One well-publicized incident happened at the Seoul Olympics in 1988 when sprinter Ben Johnson tested positive for anabolic steroids and was stripped of his gold medal. Athletes may also misuse drugs to relax, cope with stress or boost their own confidence.

Athletes may have several reasons for using performance-enhancing drugs. An athlete may want to:
- Build mass and strength of muscles and/or bones
- Increase delivery of oxygen to exercising tissues
- Mask pain
- Stimulate his or her body (increase alertness, reduce fatigue, increase aggressiveness)
- Relax
- Reduce weight
- Hide their use of other drugs

Figure 1: Classes of Performance-Enhancing Drugs

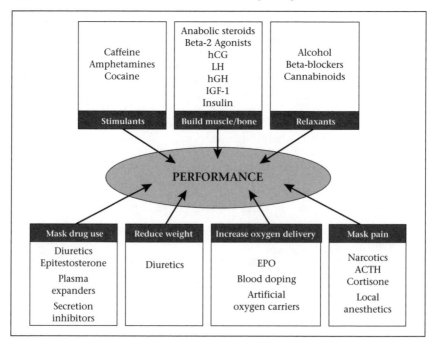

The classes of drugs used for these purposes are shown in Figure 1. Most of the drugs shown are banned outright in Olympic competitions. However, some of these drugs (cortisone, local anesthetics) are restricted in Olympic competition because they have legitimate clinical uses. We'll look at each major class of drug and tell you about the dangerous side effects.

Building mass and strength

Mass- and strength-enhancing drugs used by athletes include:
- Anabolic Steroids
- Beta-2 Agonists
- Human Chorionic Gonadotropin (hCG)
- Luteinizing Hormone (LH)
- Human Growth Hormone (hGH)
- Insulin-like Growth Factor (IGF-1)
- Insulin

Anabolic Steroids. A steroid is a chemical substance derived from cholesterol. The body has several major steroid hormones (cortisol and testosterone in the male, estrogen and progesterone in the female). Catabolic steroids break down tissue, and anabolic steroids build up tissue. Anabolic steroids build muscle and bone mass primarily by stimulating the muscle and bone cells to make new protein.

Athletes use anabolic steroids because they increase muscle strength by encouraging new muscle growth.

Athletes use anabolic steroids because they increase muscle strength by encouraging new muscle growth. Anabolic steroids are similar in structure to the male sex hormone, testosterone, so they enhance male reproductive and secondary sex characteristics (testicle development, hair growth, thickening of the vocal cords). They allow the athlete to train harder and longer at any given period.

Anabolic steroids are mostly testosterone (male sex hormone) and its derivatives (natural, artificial). Examples of anabolic steroids include:
- testosterone
- dihydrotestosterone
- androstenedione (Andro)
- dehydroepiandrosterone (DHEA)
- clostebol
- nandrolone

These substances can be injected or taken as pills.

Anabolic steroids have a number of possible and well known side effects, including:
- jaundice and liver damage because these substances are normally broken down in the liver
- mood swings, depression and aggression because they act on various centers of the brain

In males, the excessive concentrations interfere with normal sexual function and cause:

- baldness
- infertility
- breast development

In females, the excessive concentrations cause male characteristics to develop and interfere with normal female functions. The drugs can:

- stimulate hair growth on the face and body
- suppress or interfere with menstrual cycle, possibly leading to infertility
- thicken the vocal cords, which causes the voice to deepen, possibly permanently
- if pregnant, interfere with the developing fetus

Beta-2 Adrenergic Agonists. When inhaled, beta-2 agonists relax the smooth muscle in the airways of asthma patients by mimicking the actions of epinephrine and norepinephrine, substances that are secreted by sympathetic nerves. However when injected into the bloodstream, these drugs can build muscle mass (anabolic effect) and reduce body fat (catabolic effect). The anabolic effect appears to directly affect building proteins in the muscles, which is independent of nervous or cardiovascular effects. Some examples of beta-2 agonists include:

- clenbuterol
- tertbutaline (Bricanyl)
- salbutamol (Ventolin)
- fenoterol
- bambuterol

Some of these substances (Ventolin, Bricanyl) are permitted in inhaler forms with written medical consent.

The major side effects include:

- nausea, headaches and dizziness because these substances constrict blood vessels in the brain
- muscle cramps because they constrict blood vessels in muscles
- rapid heart beats or flutters because they stimulate heart rate

Human Chorionic Gonadotropin (hCG). hCG is a naturally occurring protein hormone produced by the developing fetus and detected in most home pregnancy kits. hCG stimulates the development of natural male and female sex steroids (testosterone, estrogen and progesterone). The increase in testosterone levels in males by the use of hCG would stimulate muscle development as with anabolic steroids. hCG is not banned in female athletes because it would not lead to muscle development and might naturally occur in high levels if the athlete is pregnant. The side effects of hCG in males are the same as those of anabolic steroids.

In addition to [steroids] . . . , some athletes take drugs and engage in practices that increase the amount of oxygen in tissues.

Luteinizing Hormone (LH). LH is a peptide hormone secreted by the pituitary gland at the base of the brain. LH is important for maintaining normal levels of testosterone in the male and estrogen in the female. In women, a surge of LH during mid-cycle is the signal for ovulation. In men, excess LH or artificial LH derivatives (tamoxifen) would increase testosterone levels and have the same effects as anabolic steroids. Although no general side effects exist, any possible side effects might be similar to those of anabolic steroids.

Human Growth Hormone (hGH). hGH is a naturally occurring protein hormone produced by the pituitary gland and is important for normal human growth and development, especially in children and teenagers. Low hGH levels in children and teenagers result in dwarfism. Excessive hGH levels increase muscle mass by stimulating protein synthesis, strengthen bones by stimulating bone growth and reduce body fat by stimulating the breakdown of fat cells. Use of hGH has become increasingly popular because it is difficult to detect. Side effects include:

- overgrowth of hand, feet, and face (acromegaly) because of the increased muscle and bone development in these parts.
- enlarged internal organs, especially heart, kidneys, tongue and liver.
- heart problems.

Insulin-Like Growth Factor (IGF-1). IGF-1, which is also called somatomedin-C, is a naturally occurring protein that helps in the action of hGH. It also stimulates protein synthesis and reduces fat. Excessive IGF-1 would increase muscle and bone mass as hGH does. Side effects include low blood sugar (hypoglycemia) and other side effects similar to hGH.

Other compounds, . . . can be used to reduce the presence of banned substances in blood samples.

Insulin. Insulin is a natural protein hormone produced by the pancreas, which is important for metabolism of sugars, starches, fats, and proteins. It is necessary for the treatment of juvenile (Type I) diabetes. In athletes, insulin combined with anabolic steroids or hGH could increase muscle mass by stimulating protein synthesis. Side effects are mainly low blood sugar associated with shaking, nausea and weakness, but excessive hypoglycemia can lead to coma and death.

Increasing oxygen in tissues

In addition to taking drugs that build mass and strength, some athletes take drugs and engage in practices that increase the amount of oxygen in tissues, including protein hormones, artificial oxygen carriers and blood doping.

Protein Hormones. Erythropoietin (EPO) is a naturally occurring protein hormone that is secreted by the kidneys during low oxygen conditions. EPO stimulates the bone marrow stem cells to make red blood cells, which increase the delivery of oxygen to the kidney. Endurance athletes, such as those who compete in marathons, cycling or cross-country skiing, can use EPO to increase their oxygen supply by as much as seven to 10 percent. EPO is difficult to detect. The increased red cell density (secondary polycythemia) caused by EPO, however, can thicken the blood. The thickened blood, which is more like honey than water, does not flow through the blood vessels well. To pump the thickened blood, the heart must work harder, which increases the chances of heart attack and stroke.

Artificial Oxygen Carriers. Artificial oxygen carriers are man-made substances that can do the work of hemoglobin, the oxygen-carrying protein in your blood. Doctors use them to treat breathing difficulties in premature infants, in patients with severe lung injuries and in deep-sea divers. They include substances such as perfluorocarbons, synthetic- or modified-hemoglobins and liposome-encased hemoglobins (artificial red cells). It is not clear how they benefit athletes. Possible side effects include immune problems (fever, decreased platelets, increased phagocyte counts), cardiovascular problems (high blood pressure), iron overload and kidney damage.

Blood Doping. Blood doping is the practice of infusing whole blood into an athlete in order to increase oxygen delivery to the tissues. A similar effect can be achieved by training at high altitudes. An athlete who infuses his own blood may cause infection or cardiovascular problems because of the increased blood volume (high blood pressure, blood clots, heart failure and stroke). An athlete who uses someone else's blood runs the risk of acquiring viral infections (hepatitis, HIV/AIDS).

Masking pain

Along with training and performing to be a world-class athlete comes the pain of injuries. Sometimes, athletes try to mask their injury pain with drugs, including narcotics, protein hormones, cortisone and local anesthetics (injectibles).

Narcotics. Narcotics are used to treat pain and include substances such as morphine, methadone and heroin. Narcotics are highly addictive, and the "high" associated with their use can impair mental abilities (judgment, balance and concentration). Also, athletes who continue to compete with an injury run the risk of further damage or complications.

Protein Hormones. Adrenocorticotrophic Hormone (ACTH) is a naturally occurring protein hormone that is secreted by the pituitary gland and stimulates the production of hormones from the adrenal cortex (cortisone, corticosteroids, glucocorticoids). These adrenal cortex hormones are important in reducing inflammation in injuries and allergic responses. So, by using ACTH to stimulate internal adrenal cortex hormones, an athlete could mask an injury. Possible side effects include stomach irritation, ulcers, mental irritation and long-term effects (weakening bones and muscles).

Cortisone. Cortisone is one of the adrenal cortex hormones mentioned above. Clinically, it is injected to reduce inflammation in injuries and allergic responses. The advantages and side effects of its use are the same as with ACTH.

Local Anesthetics. Local anesthetics, like those used by your dentist or doctor, are used to mask pain in the short-term without impairing mental abilities. They include novocaine, procaine, lidocaine and lignocaine. Athletes may use them so that they can continue to compete while injured. The major problem with their use is the possibility of further aggravating an injury.

Stimulants, relaxants and weight control

Many athletes live within strict social and dietary guidelines. To cope with stress, general fatigue and weight, many athletes turn to stimulating, relaxing and weight controlling drugs.

Stimulants. Stimulants are generally used to help athletes stay alert, reduce fatigue and maintain aggressiveness. They act on the body to make the heart beat faster, the lungs breathe faster and the brain work faster. Stimulants include caffeine, amphetamines, ephedrine, phenylephrine, phenylproanolamine, strychnine and cocaine. Possible side effects include nervousness, shaking, irregular heartbeats, high blood pressure, convulsions and even sudden death.

There will be a constant struggle between the development/use of new drugs for performance enhancement and of new tests to detect these drugs.

Relaxants. Relaxants come in various forms, including alcohol, prescriptions such as beta-blockers, and cannabinoids such as marijuana.

- Alcohol is commonly used to help people relax because it reduces activity in the brain and nervous system. While it may help an athlete relax and cope with the pressures of competition, it can also significantly impair mental functions (judgment, balance, coordination). It is restricted in the Olympics and banned altogether in certain events.
- Beta-blockers are commonly prescribed to treat high blood pressure by causing the heart to slow down and blood vessels to relax. Athletes who require steady hands in competition, such as those competing in archery or shooting events, may use them. Possible side effects include lower than normal blood pressure (hypotension), slow heart rate and fatigue.
- Cannabinoids, mainly marijuana and hashish, have no clinical value, but have recently been used for relieving pain in terminally ill cancer patients. Cannabinoids cause hallucinations, induce drowsiness, increase the heart rate and impair mental functions (judgment, balance, coordination and memory).

Weight Control. Diuretics are commonly prescribed to treat high blood pressure and are often found in diet pills. Diuretics act on the kidney to increase the flow of urine. Diuretics include furosemide, acetazolamide, bumetanide and ethacrynic acid. They are used by athletes whose events have weight restrictions (weightlifting, rowing, horse racing). Diuretics are also used to mask the use of other drugs. Because they increase the amount of urine produced, they dilute the concentration of other drugs in the urine. Possible side effects include dehydration, dizziness, cramps, heart damage and kidney failure.

Masking drug use

As previously mentioned, diuretics can be used to reduce the presence of drugs in urine samples. Other compounds, including Epitestosterone, plasma expanders and secretion inhibitors, can be used to reduce the presence of banned substances in blood samples.

Epitestosterone. Epitestosterone is a biological form of testosterone that does not enhance performance. Drug tests for testosterone typically measure the ratio of testosterone to epitestosterone (T/E ratio). An athlete can inject epitestosterone, lower the T/E ratio and hide the use of testosterone. By itself, epitestosterone has no real harmful side effects.

Plasma Expanders. Plasma expanders are substances that are used to increase the fluid component of blood. They are used to treat victims of shock, trauma and surgery. They include Albumex, Gelofusine and Haemaccel. Athletes can use these substances to dilute the concentration of banned substances (EPO) in their blood. Most side effects include moderate to severe allergic reactions.

Secretion Inhibitors. Many drugs and foreign substances have structures that are shaped like organic acids. In the body, these organic acids are removed by a protein in the kidney that transports organic acids. If this protein can be blocked, then these drugs or foreign substances would not appear in the urine. These inhibitors include probenecid, sulfinpyrazone and related compounds. Doctors use these inhibitors to treat gout. However, the drugs can be used to manipulate the results of urine drug tests. Possible side effects include nausea, vomiting, allergic reactions and kidney problems.

Testing athletes for drug use

The majority of drugs that can be used by athletes can be detected in samples of urine. An athlete is told by a drug control officer to submit a urine sample for testing. The sample is then sent to a laboratory for analysis and the results are reported back to the governing athletic agency. For some substances, blood samples may be required.

Gas Chromatography/Mass Spectrometry. Gas chromatography and mass spectrometry are the most common methods of chemical analysis. These tests can be done on urine and blood samples. In gas chromatography, the sample is vaporized in the presence of a gaseous solvent and placed through a long path of a machine. Each substance dissolves differently in the gas and stays in the gas phase for a unique, specific time (retention time). Typically the substance comes out of the gas and is absorbed on to a solid or liquid, which is then analyzed by a detector. When the sample is analyzed, the retention time is reported or plotted (chromatogram). Standard samples of drugs are run, as well as the urine/blood samples, so that specific drugs can be identified and quantified in the chromatograms of the urine/blood samples.

In mass spectrometry, samples are blown apart with an electron beam and the fragments are accelerated down a long magnetic tube to a detector. Each substance has a unique "fingerprint" in the mass spectrometer. Again, standard samples are run for identification and quantification of drugs in the urine/blood samples.

Immuno-Assays. Some substances (such as hCG, LH, ACTH) can be measured in urine samples using an immuno-assay. In this test, the sample is mixed with a solution containing an antibody specific to the tested substance. An antibody is a protein that binds only a specific substance and is how the body recognizes foreign substances. The antibody in the test is usually tagged with a fluorescent dye or radioactive substance. The amount of fluorescent light or radioactivity is measured and is related to the concentration of the tested substance in the sample.

Tests Under Development. Currently, there are no reliable tests for hGH, IGF-1 and EPO. However, a test for EPO is being developed.* The EPO test looks at the size of red blood cells. It has been noticed that synthetic EPO produces red blood cells that are smaller and bind more iron then natural EPO. So, the size and iron content of red blood cells from a blood sample are analyzed to determine whether an athlete has used EPO.

It seems that drug testing will become an integral part of sports competitions. There will a constant struggle between the development/use of new drugs for performance enhancement and of new tests to detect these drugs.

*[Editor's note: A test for EPO was developed in August 2000 and adopted by the International Olympic Committee (IOC). New forms of EPO being used by athletes may render the current test obsolete.]

2

Athletes Will Never Stop Using Performance- Enhancing Drugs

Matt Barnard

Matt Barnard writes for the New Statesman, *a news magazine.*

The moral crusade against the use of performance-enhancing drugs in sports is being waged by international athletic associations and their corporate sponsors, who publicly maintain that drugs violate the moral borders of clean athletic competition. However, in their quest for fans and profits, these organizations covertly encourage drug use by demanding ever higher standards of achievement from athletes, only to condemn the few athletes who get caught. Fans, on the other hand, have demonstrated a willingness to support drug-aided athletes like major league baseball player Mark McGwire, who broke the home run record in 1998 while admitting steroid use. It is time to recognize that the use of performance-enhancing drugs is here to stay and that elite athletes will go to extreme lengths to succeed.

Florence Griffith Joyner ("Flo-Jo") died, aged 38, from heart seizure in September 1998. Even before her untimely death, the shadow of suspicion hung over her glorious two gold medals and one silver at the Seoul Olympics in 1988: with her muscular form and husky voice typical of steroid users, and with her retirement announced abruptly in 1989, when mandatory random testing for drugs was introduced, there were whispers that Flo-Jo had used performance-enhancing drugs.

Spotlighting the debate

Flo-Jo's death will throw the spotlight back on to the debate over drugs in sports. In early September 1998, another athlete was etching his name into the record books. The US baseball player Mark McGwire hit the most home runs ever in a single season, America's most prestigious sporting record. He is the first athlete in history to break a record while publicly admitting his use of performance-enhancing drugs. McGwire has admitted taking the drug androstenedione, which helps to build muscle and aids recovery from injury or exhaustion. The drug is on the banned list of the International Olympic Committee (IOC) but is not banned by baseball's governing body, nor is it illegal. So far the use of drugs has not doomed baseball.

McGwire's chemically-aided race against the record book is credited with reviving interest in America's first game, giving it a renewed sense of value after the player strikes of 1994. As in many walks of life, unbridled success is able to sweep any latent moral misgivings neatly under the carpet.

Less predictably, however, the crowds lining the roads during the 1998 Tour de France applauded the cyclists as they swept past, supporting them despite the revelations of systematic drug-taking. The heavy-handed way the authorities conducted their investigation did little to win them support, and many spectators found it easy to empathise with athletes who had spent eight hours a day for two-and-a-half weeks slogging their guts out in one of the world's toughest competitions.

The moral crusade against the use of drugs in sport, like most moral crusades, is surrounded by myth.

The moral crusade against the use of drugs in sport, like most moral crusades, is surrounded by myth. One of the myths is that fans won't pay to see drug-aided athletes perform, something that McGwire's example, and to a lesser degree the Tour de France, seem directly to contradict. It is said that more people turn up to watch McGwire warm up than attend most matches.

A second myth is that using drugs means that athletes don't have to work for their achievements. But, as Nicholas Pierce, lecturer in sport and exercise medicine at Queen's Medical Centre in Nottingham, comments: "Athletes will always be pushing themselves to the limit; if you could help push them further, they will go further."

The former cyclist Tommy Simpson is often mentioned in the context of sport and drugs, as he was one of the first athletes to die as a result of taking performance-enhancing stimulants. What commentators tend not to mention is that he literally worked himself to death. He pushed himself so hard that his heart gave out. Whatever one thinks about athletes who take drugs, they don't lack courage.

It is undoubtedly true, nonetheless, that the idea of using performance-enhancing drugs is deeply disturbing to a great many people. John Whetton is a former Olympic 1,500 metres finalist and European champion and is now a principal lecturer in life sciences at Nottingham Trent University. He is very clear that chemicals and sport shouldn't mix: "Using chemicals to do what your body isn't capable of doing is cheating, but it is a form of cheating that is hidden and therefore it is a nasty form of cheating."

But McGwire is open about his drug-taking, and as has become clear in the aftermath of the 1998 Tour, within cycling the use of drugs is an open secret.

Keeping sports "natural"

Yet why are athletes who secretly do altitude training not tarred with the same brush? Clearly, the opposition to using drugs in sport is based on more fundamental assumptions than that it is simply not allowed by the rules.

From the time the Greeks formulated the Olympic ideal, sport has held a more significant place in our culture than merely a leisure pursuit. In many ways it is used as a looking glass for the way we think about society. Richard Kerridge, co-editor of *Writing the Environment,* published in 1998, sees society's attitude to sport as being a web of concepts all entangled around the idea of what is "natural" and how we define "nature."

We see sport, he believes, as a celebration of nature, a way of demonstrating the wonders of creation, which is combined with the idea of discipline, abstinence and purity. "In part," he says, "it's to do with the Christian tradition, in which to violate the laws of nature is to usurp the power of God. The taboo is about interfering in nature and interfering with the body." With such a background, it is not surprising that drugs are anathema.

On top of those ancient foundations is the more recent idea that sport is a form of capitalist competition. Kerridge says: "Characteristic of this attitude is that sport involves a relentless pressure for a kind of growth, so the standards always have to be pushed higher and higher."

Though capitalism is based on the dog-eat-dog world of Darwinian survival, historians point out that the tradition of economic liberalism has always been combined with a strong sense of moral paternalism. It is perfectly acceptable to have obscene differences in wealth, but if a pauper is caught stealing a loaf of bread they should be publicly flogged. Similarly in sport, athletes and sporting nations may have hugely differing resources and expertise, but that is part of the free market of sport. However, that free market has strict moral borders, and drug-taking falls outside them.

Many feel that sporting bodies and sponsors covertly encourage athletes to take drugs, yet abandon and condemn the few who get caught.

In order to reinforce that border, everyone involved in the "war on drugs" emphasises the physical risks involved. They are significant: liver failure and an increased chance of a heart attack are among the conditions associated with performance-enhancing drugs. Because of the ban on them, however, very little research has been done on how to reduce the risk.

The former Soviet states poured millions of pounds into developing performance-enhancing drugs, using the athlete as guinea pig—the individual as the servant of the collective. Nicholas Pierce is completely opposed to the use of drugs in sport, but is forced to admit that with very large funds available it would be possible to develop a performance-enhancing drug that is virtually free of side-effects. And that, he argues, would have beneficial consequences for the rest of society: "It would be a tremendous boost for medicine as well. It would help people recover from operations and all sorts of things."

Covert encouragement from sponsors

Athletes would become the equivalent of test pilots, who take high risks and sometimes get injured or killed. Unlike test pilots, though, at present there would be no safety checks or organisations to back them up. Indeed, many feel that sporting bodies and sponsors covertly encourage athletes to take drugs, yet abandon and condemn the few who get caught.

Michelle Verroken, head of the Ethics and Doping Directorate at the UK Sports Council, has had direct experience of the lengths to which sports bodies will go to protect themselves. "It's not unusual," she says, "to have some of the major sporting organisations in this country asking us not to test athletes prior to a major sporting event like the Olympic or Commonwealth games."

Verroken, like many others, also raises questions about the drug-testing at the 1996 Atlanta Olympics, where the results went through organisations that had a direct interest in making sure the games were a commercial success, rather than through an independent testing organisation.

"In Euro 96, the Union des Associations Européennes de Football (UEFA) worked very closely with us, so all the reports from the drug-testing process were reported through us. Is that what happened in Atlanta, or were the reports going straight back into the hands of the sports bodies who have a vested interest in making sure nothing clouds that event?

"It's not just an organisation like the International Olympic Committee, but it may be the organising committee from Atlanta or sponsors who pay an awful lot of money to have their name associated with the event and suddenly they are the 'whatever-company drug-infested games.' Those are the sorts of headlines that devastate the marketing people. Athletes feel they have been badly let down by the sports organisations that should have been protecting them."

One of the most surprising reactions to McGwire's achievement of breaking the record for home runs came from one of his teammates, who said: "What Mark has is God-given." It seems that in baseball the competitors have accepted that drug-taking is a legitimate training aid, but that it is only an aid.

Drugs are here to stay

The truth is that drugs are here to stay. Juan Antonio Samaranch, [former] president of the IOC, had to backpedal after he said that only drugs that harmed an athlete should remain on the banned list. But his was the first official brick to fall from the dam. We will accept drugs in sport—at elite level—just as surely as we accept them in medicine, cosmetics or farming.

Verroken's response to such an assertion is simple: "If a safe performance-enhancing drug improved everybody's performance to the same extent, what would be the point of taking it?" The answer is that, rightly or wrongly, every athlete has inscribed on their heart the words *citius altius fortius*—swifter, higher, stronger, as the Olympic motto reads. They will go to almost any lengths to push the barriers back.

3

Athletes Must Stop Using Performance-Enhancing Drugs

Merrell Noden

Merrell Noden is a regular contributor to Sports Illustrated *and the author of* Home Run Heroes: Mark McGwire, Sammy Sosa, and a Season for the Ages.

The sport of track and field has been tarnished by the use of performance-enhancing drugs among its leading competitors. Each new world record raises suspicions that the record-breaker was using steroids or other performance-enhancing drugs. To reduce the temptation among athletes to use drugs and foster more realistic expectations from fans, competition should be emphasized over record-breaking as the measure of an exciting track meet. Reliable drug testing must also be put into effect to further deter athletes from using drugs.

I don't remember when I first heard about steroids. Probably it was around 1972, when they were first banned by the International Olympic Committee (IOC) and I was on the track team in high school. If there was a debate about steroids in the papers, I didn't pay much attention to it, mostly, I suspect, because I didn't think they bore relevance to my life as an athlete. I considered them the province of weightlifters, shot-putters, football players and other "big" athletes—not skinny distance runners like me.

This I do remember: I passed the summer of 1981 in a state of giddy transport, and from that I conclude that I cannot have known much about steroids yet. That was the summer Steve Ovett and Seb Coe snatched the world mile record back and forth like a couple of kids fighting over candy. By then I was teaching junior high English at Princeton Day School, and most mornings that summer my fellow teacher and running partner Eamon Downey and I would drive to a nearby deli for coffee and *The New York Times*. Every day, it seemed—though, of course, this was not literally true—one of the two Brits, each so charismatic in his own way, had run some stunning time: if not a world record, then something very close to it. For runners like Eamon and me, it was the equivalent of reading that men had walked on the moon. Anything seemed possible.

A great ugly cloud

I've lost the capacity for that sort of exhilaration. Summer 1998's unsurprising revelations of drug use among riders in the Tour de France and alleged drug-sample tampering by Irish swimmer Michelle Smith, and the bans of two U.S. track and field stars, sprinter Dennis Mitchell and shotputter Randy Barnes, felt more like deja vu than shock. My capacity for wonder has slipped away gradually over the years, starting in 1983, when I learned that steroids would also help skinny distance runners like me. If our bodies could tolerate two hard track sessions a week without steroids, we would probably be able to handle three or four with them. Sure enough, at the 1984 Olympics, one of those skinny distance runners, Martti Vainio of Finland, tested positive for steroids after finishing second in the 10,000 meters.

The use of . . . performance-enhancing drugs has covered [track and field] with a great ugly cloud.

The use of steroids and other performance-enhancing drugs has covered the sport with a great ugly cloud. At the 1992 U.S. Olympic Trials in New Orleans, when the Supreme Court granted Butch Reynolds a temporary restraining order allowing him to compete despite an earlier positive drug test, for which he had been banned for two years, I asked a respected track and field journalist, a former athlete, if he thought Reynolds was guilty. "I have no idea, but I suspect so," he said. "Why? Forty-three twenty-nine." He was referring to Reynolds's world record of 43.29 seconds in the 400 meters, a time .57 of a second faster than anyone else had ever run.

And there, in a nutshell, is the awful bind that track fans find themselves in: Any dazzling world record instantly raises the specter of cheating. Whatever miraculous feats I may witness in the future—a man longjumping 30 feet, a woman running a four-minute mile—I doubt I'll shake off the conviction that those marks have not been achieved naturally.

This sorry state is not the fault solely of athletes, most of whom, I think, would love to see a return to the level playing field of the presteroid era. But where's the incentive? Meet promoters sell tickets based on the promise of records; agents make more money as their athletes run faster or jump higher; federation officials obtain sponsorship based on how hot their sport is. The last thing these people want is a scandal. That's why Olympic officials trumpeted the fact that of the 1,800 drug tests conducted at the Atlanta Games, only two were positive. It's great p.r.; it's what we all want to hear.

A 70-foot-plus shot-putter once told me that he believed no one had ever thrown 70 feet without an artificial boost; the human body just isn't built to do that any more than it's built to race over the Alps day after day on a bicycle. So imagine yourself a young shot-putter, in love with your event. Do you stay clean and top out at, say, 66 feet, never having reached the glorious European circuit, beaten meet after meet by guys you're sure are juiced? Virtue may be its own reward, but if you're willing to be honest, I think you'll agree that's not an easy decision.

Several decades of . . . virtually meaningless [drug] testing opened a Pandora's box of artificially boosted performances that raised fans' expectations.

Unfortunately, several decades of, first, no testing and then virtually meaningless testing opened a Pandora's box of artificially boosted performances that raised fans' expectations. A few years ago I stood in Stanford Stadium with discus thrower John Powell. He pointed to the huge, empty stands surrounding us and reminded me that he had seen them full for one of the U.S.-U.S.S.R. dual meets in the early 1960s. "Would all those people come out again to watch sprinters run 10.2?" he asked.

Fixing the mess

How do we fix this mess? Here are two suggestions that might offer a first step.

First, since human evolution can't keep pace with our hunger for new records, and neither can advances in training, why not reemphasize competition over records? Who can actually see the difference between a 9.84 100 and a 10.04 100? But a close race, with two or three athletes straining toward the finish, now, that's exciting. Admittedly, reeducating the public to look at track and field this way would be hard, especially when seemingly everyone—TV commentators, meet promoters, this magazine—regards records as the measure of a great meet.

Second, I'm convinced that the best hope for cleaning this up lies with the athletes. Drug testing that is planned and enforced by nonathlete administrators feels imposed, inviting attempts to circumvent it. Several decades ago Coe and current USA Track & Field CEO Craig Masback, then an outstanding miler, pushed for the formation of a track and field athletes' union. It didn't happen, largely because of the difficulties of uniting competitors from so many countries and so many events. The time has come to try again, and meaningful, reliable drug testing should be the body's first order of business.

Although Ben Johnson's stanozolol-fueled 9.79 in the 100 at the Seoul Olympics is one of just a handful of world records to have been thrown out because of a positive drug test, there is no question that other world marks have been set by athletes using steroids or other illicit performance enhancers. Haven't those record setters forced their rivals—and athletes of the future—to use drugs too? It's that or chase fruitlessly after marks that won't be broken by clean athletes.

Tom Tellez, Carl Lewis's great coach, told me that he does not think Lewis could ever have equaled the 9.79 Johnson ran in Seoul, and the current world record, the 9.84 that Donovan Bailey ran at the Atlanta Games, is still a long way from Johnson's discredited mark. Had Johnson not tested positive, how long would we have had to wait for someone even to approach the 100 record?

If a sprinter ever does run a 9.79, of course, fans will automatically assume that he has been using performance-enhancing drugs, whether he has or not. Is that the legacy today's track and field athletes want to leave behind? Cynicism where there might be exhilaration?

Any dazzling world record instantly raises the specter of cheating.

4

Performance-Enhancing Drugs Tarnish Athletics

European Commission

*The European Commission is the executive body responsible for imple-
menting the legislation adopted by the Parliament and Council of the
European Union. The commission enforces the European Union's policy
banning performance-enhancing drugs from athletic competition.*

"Doping" is the illegal misuse of drugs by athletes to enhance performance when training or participating in a sporting event.
While athletes have used plants and other substances to artificially enhance performance throughout history, dangerous doping methods are now commonplace. Some athletes view doping as
the only way to keep up with the fierce demands of athletic competition. In addition to jeopardizing public health, doping is at
odds with the principle that athletes should work without artificial resources to achieve success. Education and prevention cam-
paigns must be undertaken to stamp out doping.

What does doping really mean? One way of finding out is to look in
the dictionary, where it tells you that it comes from a Dutch word
"doop" meaning a thick liquid or sauce, a reminder that it originally referred to a South African drink. In days gone by, "dope" was something
you drank to help you work hard, if only for a short space of time. So, in
English, "to dope" means to administer a drug, specifically as a stimulant.

Artificially enhancing performance

An official definition of "doping" was adopted in Uriarge in 1963. Since
then, it has meant the use of substances and any other available methods
of artificially enhancing performance in a sporting event, or when prepar-
ing for it, in a way which violates sporting ethics and damages the physical and psychological health of the athlete or player.

So doping is an operation which sets out quite deliberately and knowingly to do two things: combat fatigue and enhance performance.

From "Joining Forces Against Doping—What Is Doping?" by the European Commission,
http://europa.eu.int.

This definition needs some refining. To start with, there are the medical aspects.

What doping involves is misusing medicinal products or techniques. Where products are concerned, it can mean every drug in the pharmacopoeia. Some of them are exogenous, which means coming from outside the body and therefore easy to identify. Others are endogenous, stimulating the body to secrete particular molecules itself. Identifying these means doing medical tests. When it comes to techniques, it boils down to using medical practices for the wrong purposes, e.g. the practice of putting sportsmen and women on [intravenous] drips [to replace lost body fluids during athletic events].

We also have to find a definition of doping in terms of the law. It flies in the face of sporting ethics, and tarnishes the image of sport as a means of keeping society in balance. Doping is also bad for the health. It is a criminal offence, and both users and suppliers of "dope" can be punished.

[Doping] flies in the face of sporting ethics, and tarnishes the image of sport as a means of keeping society in balance.

And then, of course, there is the definition of the term as understood by sportspeople themselves. More and more they seem to be split between two camps. For some, there is no "doping" unless a person's life is in danger. They can accept a situation where drugs are administered by a doctor or under medical supervision. Others use the term to mean engaging in practices or taking substances which are against the rules. The problem here arises from the lack of uniform standards. The criteria for regarding products as forbidden drugs vary from one sport to another, as the list drawn up by the International Olympic Committee (IOC) is not yet universally accepted.

The history of doping

Higher, faster, stronger—that was the Olympic motto dreamed up by Baron Pierre de Coubertin at the end of the 19th century. Yet men and women have always striven to excel themselves and sport, or physical exercise in the broader sense, has given them the opportunity to do so. And there have always been techniques for sportspeople to apply or substances to take to increase their strength, raise their standard or improve their performance artificially. The poppy was already being used in the Neolithic era, and opium was highly prized by the Egyptians, the Romans and, of course, the Greeks, who were also especially fond of beef when the Games were on, believing that it gave them the strength of ten. Both then and subsequently, in other parts of the world, ginseng root, coca leaves, hemp, maté and kava (an extract of the pepper plant) were also highly valued.

Doping, however, in the sense used today, really came onto the scene in the 19th century. In a way it was brought into being by medical advances and by the emergence of sport as we see it today.

The first drugs to be used were heroin and morphine. Heroin was mainly found in horse-racing circles, while morphine was very much in fashion in boxing and so-called endurance sports. At any rate it was suspected of having caused the death of Arthur Lindon, a Welsh racing cyclist who died a few months after the Bordeaux-Paris race of 1896, thereby becoming the first ever recorded victim of doping.

Things really got out of hand at the beginning of the 20th century, with strychnine and ephedrine making their appearance, not to mention steroids.

The team behind Thomas Hicks, a runner who won the marathon at the 1904 London Olympics, were clearly giving him the first of these, laced with alcohol and cocaine, to push him to victory.

The second (ephedrine) was actually the forerunner of amphetamines. Developed at the beginning of the 1930s, amphetamines first came into use in sport at the Berlin Olympics in 1936. They were widely used in battle in the Second World War and became extremely popular in the years that followed. What made them especially common was that most of the time they could be bought freely. Some time later, however, they were clearly implicated in at least three deaths. The victims were two cyclists, Knut Enemark Jensen from Denmark, during the 100 kilometre race against the clock at the Rome Olympics in 1960, and Tom Simpson of England in the Tour de France in 1967, as well as a French footballer, Jean-Louis Quadri, who died in 1968.

Hormone doping arose out of the work done as long ago as 1889 by a French physiologist, Edouard Brown-Séquard, and then in 1935 by Ernest Laqueur, who isolated the male hormone, testosterone. Four years later the Wolverhampton football team tried it out in England. It was not until the 1950s, though, that anabolic steroids really made their entry onto the sporting stage, starting with weight-lifting and athletics. But they spread fast. The Spanish tennis player Andres Gimeno admitted taking them in 1959, a long time before it was discovered what lay behind East Germany's sporting successes in the 1970s or before the Canadian sprinter Ben Johnson was disqualified from the Olympic Games in Seoul in 1988.

Over the last few years, doping has taken a new and dangerous turn. Growth hormones have appeared, as well as intravenous doping involving transfusions of the athlete's own blood, and then erythropoietin (EPO), perfluorcarbons and reticulate haemoglobin. In none of these cases has respect for human life necessarily been the primary consideration.

All this has changed the whole course of doping. Drugs used to be taken just for a one-off effect which activated various standard bodily functions, but now they may bring about the biological reprogramming of the body. To put it plainly, the time is not far off when it will be scientifically possible to make artificial but lasting changes in the way an organ functions and when the technicians of sport will be able to tailor each drug to meet the specifications for a particular level of performance.

The Festina affair

The skies over Dublin were changeable. Everything was ready for the 1998 Tour de France to set off from Ireland, and France had not yet won the World Cup. A few hours before the cyclists were to leave the starting line for the most prestigious cycle race of the season, a strange rumour began to spread. In the middle of the week a trainer for the Festina team—the pick of the bunch, the team featuring such riders as Richard Virenque, the darling of the French public, world champion Laurent Brochard and Alex Zulle, twice winner of the Tour of Spain—was checked by customs at Neuville-en-Ferrain on the French-Belgian border. And according to the rumour, the officers had found a great many unusual things in his vehicle, which was officially accredited to the Tour de France. Shortly afterwards the world was to learn that he had been carrying EPO, growth hormones, testosterone, corticoids, amphetamines and vaccines.

At the Tour, they started to shake in their shoes. For the first time in the history of the Tour and for the first time, indeed, in the history of cycle-racing and sport, the participants realised that the authorities were aware of how little winning the race had to do with sporting prowess alone and had decided to do something about the doping.

But it was a bitter struggle. When the Tour got started in Dublin, the Festina affair had still got no further than merely questioning the Festina team's trainer, Willy Voet. Not until he confessed on 14 July and Bruno Rossel and Eric Ryckaert, the team's manager and doctor, were detained for questioning did people at last realise that in this particular case the doping operation had been run by a very well-oiled and experienced machine.

The Festina affair began to have wider ramifications. On 17 July, Festina's cyclists were disqualified from the Tour. Another case came to light when investigations were started into the Dutch TVM team in Rheims, and the Tour only made it to Paris a fortnight later by the skin of its teeth. Twice, on 24 and 29 July, the participants threatened to go on strike. Some teams had their vehicles and hotel rooms searched. On police orders riders were made to take medical tests. One of them, Rodolfo Massi, was placed under investigation, as was Nicolas Terrados, the doctor for the Once team, a Spanish line-up which withdrew from the Tour along with five others.

At the end of the day, when Marco Pantani, the first Italian to wear the winner's yellow jersey since Felice Gimondi in 1965, crossed the finishing line in Paris at the head of the pack, everyone was left with a strange taste in the mouth. For once it had become abundantly clear how widespread doping was in sport.

Sportsmen and women are . . . acting under pressure from an environment which practically makes doping essential.

And then the fight began. It was a hard battle. Some called for all sport to be completely above board, while others argued that there was a place for doping provided it was done under medical supervision and did not jeopardise the health of the competitor concerned. Some saw sport as a school for human behaviour, while others, themselves active sportsmen and women, were not at all keen to break with old habits.

It was a very real conflict, fought out on the sports field, with the organisers of the Tour de France putting the ethics of cycling at the top of their list of concerns. And there it stayed when the International Olympic Committee, at the beginning of February 1999, held an anti-doping conference and set up the World Anti-Doping Agency whose primary task was to make sure that the Sydney Olympics were clean.

It cannot be right . . . to treat doping as respectable just because it is common practice in the society we live in.

Governments were also involved. On the initiative of Marie-George Buffet, the Minister for Youth and Sport, France passed a new law on action to combat doping. This made safeguarding the health of sportsmen and women the main priority, stressed the need for prevention and laid down stiffer penalties for suppliers. Things began moving in other European countries as well. When, in May, the French courts again looked into the habits and practices of the cycling fraternity, the Italian courts (especially those in Bologna and Turin), not wanting to be left behind, began investigating cases in a variety of sports, including football and cycling. The Italian Minister for Sport, Giovanna Melandrini, said she was determined to move in the same direction as Marie-George Buffet. And lastly, as the German courts looked into what had happened in the world of East German sport, the European Union's Ministers for Sport said they were anxious to be involved in the Anti-Doping Agency set up by the IOC.

The challenge to sport and the media

With sport operating as an organised system for producing performances, there is a built-in tendency to stray from the straight and narrow. The task for sportsmen or women, especially in the top rank, is to beat the others and get a result. This twofold imperative creates a third one: they have to equip themselves to achieve their aims. So, to their way of thinking, doping does not seem like cheating; to put it bluntly, it is just something that has to be done.

The system makes increasingly gruelling demands on its practitioners and they have to keep up. Sporting calendars are getting fuller and fuller.

Sportsmen also have to keep up with a system which is making top-flight athletes and players more and more frail and tired. They now have to cope with ever tighter constraints imposed by the media and with economic necessities which are more and more pressing every day. In these circumstances the decision to take drugs is often taken passively. Sportsmen and women are, in a sense, acting under pressure from an environment which practically makes doping essential.

In the broader context, however, we need to stress that this need to resort to artificial ways of carrying off a performance is at odds with the basic values of sport as a social, cultural and educational activity. On the principle that all athletes and players contain within themselves the resources they need to bring out their personal best, doping diverts sport away from its true purpose. It prevents it from being a school for human behaviour.

The media influence sport in two ways. Firstly, they turn ordinary happenings into "events" and even set about making sure there are more of them, for essentially economic motives. Secondly, in some cases the media are well on the way to making organisers follow *their* rules. Sport no longer just means physical exercise. Since the end of the 1970s, and especially since the media began to call the tune, it has been turning into show-business, and the financial stakes involved are high. By their very essence, because they involve such huge sums of money and because of the thinking which motivates the people who organise them, these show-business events are more than likely to influence the use of drugs for doping.

The challenge to public health and medicine

Doping is a genuine public-health problem, since it affects everyone involved in sport, including amateurs and young people. All of them want to be recognised, and all of them want to identify with an élite.

What makes doping a really burning question is that the products and methods used are getting more and more dangerous and the ways they are used can easily lead to real dependence, which in the end is tantamount to drug addiction.

But prevention is no easy task. To begin with, as there are no reliable health indicators it is impossible to work out exactly how many people are affected. And it is not at all easy even today to pinpoint what the actual pathological consequences of doping are.

This means that the battle has to be waged on two fronts. First, we need to do something about prevention, in other words a public-information campaign should be directed at users and a public-education campaign at non-users. Then we need to run a public-health alertness exercise. At all times we should remember that there is a price to be paid for stamping out doping.

Athletes and players have to be kept under medical supervision. This was true before and it is still true today, for the function of medicine is to cure. Why it was overlooked before, and what makes it even more important today, is that doctors have to be concerned for the bodily and/or psychological wellbeing of the sportsmen or women under their care.

Sports medicine can almost be regarded nowadays as a kind of occupational medicine, for it, too, helps individuals adapt to a particular environment. To put it simply, with the passage of time doctors have steadily become more and more involved in bringing athletes to the top of their form. This is obviously different from using drugs to enhance performance. And that is where the borderline lies between what is known as "medical preparation" and doping.

We need a code of practice for doctors to follow, and the resources to put it into effect. For there are now real dilemmas facing the medical profession. Refusing to take part in doping means, as far as doctors are concerned, not just objecting to the prescribing of banned products, but also rejecting the use of authorised substances which are administered in ways or prescribed in doses incompatible with medical ethics or sporting ethics.

But to push this line of reasoning to its limits, and looking at the way things are developing today, might a doctor who refuses to take part in doping eventually be suspected of refusing to give help to a person at risk?

The challenge to society

Obviously, sport is not the only sphere of human activity where drugs are used. There are other fields where rivalry and competition sometimes push people to use artificial, i.e. chemical, means of achieving their ends.

It cannot be right, though, to treat doping as respectable just because it is common practice in the society we live in. Sport is, first and foremost, an activity unlike any other, one which relies on rules which are not supposed to be open to dispute and must be respected. Drug use for purposes other than sport as such may be dictated by the need for high performance but that does not mean the law is blind to it. There are rules governing the taking of drugs, and most cases of drug dependence arise from attempts to cure an underlying condition.

5

The Ban on Performance-Enhancing Drugs Should Continue

Economist

The Economist *is a weekly magazine covering economic and world events from around the world.*

The use of performance-enhancing drugs is widespread in Olympic sporting events like track and field and swimming. While testing procedures to catch drug cheats have become more precise and intrusive, athletes have grown more skilled at beating the tests with help from savvy medical advisers. Skeptics maintain that drug testing in sports is an exercise in futility. They contend that performance-enhancing drugs are just another way of gaining an advantage in an inherently unfair activity. In addition, they argue that such drugs should be legalized and officially regulated. However, legalizing the use of performance-enhancing drugs would turn athletes into guinea pigs and send the wrong message to impressionable children.

It was a flash of sporting brilliance. The muscle-bound, shaven-headed sprinter, born in Jamaica but wearing the colours of Canada, rose explosively from the starting blocks; 100 metres and 9.79 seconds later he raised his index finger in arrogant triumph. Ben Johnson, competing at the 1988 Seoul Olympics, had become the world's fastest man.

Within hours he had also become, for many, its most reviled. Mr Johnson, the doctors reported, had failed a drugs test. As he slunk from the Olympic village in disgrace, the second-placed Carl Lewis, from America, stepped forward to take the gold medal. Mr Johnson's humiliation, said the sporting authorities, was proof that sport will not tolerate performance-enhancing drugs.

They chant the same mantra today. The list of banned substances is like the inventory of a pharmacy. Athletes are tested in season and out of season, at random and with notice, at home and abroad. Indeed, the sensible athlete is wary even of an over-the-counter remedy for the common cold. Fail a drugs test and the punishment is a ban from competition (usually for four years, sometimes for life), which means a loss of both honour and livelihood. No wonder, given such vigilance and such penalties, the Atlanta Olympics in 1996 were declared the "cleanest" ever, with just two of the 2,000 athletes checked (out of a total 11,000 competing) failing a drugs test.

But were the Atlanta games really the cleanest ever? There are two extreme, and irreconcilable, claims made about the use of drugs in sport. The first is that drug use is rare: witness the Atlanta test results. The second is that it is ubiquitous because the cheats—or rather their doctors and chemists—are too clever for the testers. Successful cheats by definition are not caught (and are unlikely to confess). So neither claim can be proved or disproved.

What seems clear, however, is that the use of performance-enhancing drugs is a problem mainly for the athletes of track, field and swimming pool. True, some goliaths of rugby and American football have sought the help of banned body-building substances. Lyle Alzado, a former defensive lineman for the Los Angeles Raiders, died in 1992 from a rare cancer that he attributed to his prolonged use of steroids and human growth hormone. But in sports such as soccer, cricket or tennis, drug-abuse tends to be merely recreational—and thus performance-diminishing rather than enhancing.

There are several reasons why track, field and swimming are most open to cheating with drugs. Swimmers and the athletes of track and field are inherently more reliant on their physique than any ball-player. It is impossible to be a successful shotputter or weightlifter without a certain amount of sheer muscle. But it is entirely possible, as France 98 [the soccer World Cup] will prove, for successful soccer players to be skinny wraiths or squat bundles of energy: what counts are ball skills and tactical expertise that no drug can provide.

Another reason is that in team sports such as soccer and rugby an individual's weaknesses are not so exposed as they are in swimming or athletics, where even relay races in essence pit one person against another.

Sport's problem with drugs is greater than it cares to admit.

Finally, the culture of competition and imitation is strongest in track, field and swimming. If coming second is coming nowhere, as all sportspeople tend to be taught (remember the words of [football coach] Mr Lombardi), then this is most true in those individual sports where careers tend to be brief, and opportunities to win fewest. For these athletes, taking a banned drug to come first no longer seems unthinkable—particularly if those already coming first are believed to be using such a drug.

An instructive article last year in America's *Sports Illustrated* magazine referred to a 1995 survey by Bob Goldman, a Chicago doctor. Dr Goldman asked 198 American athletes of Olympic standard if, in the knowledge that they would win and would not be caught, they would take a banned substance. Only three said they would not take the drug. Dr Goldman then changed the question: by taking the drug, the athlete would win every competition for the next five years, would not be caught—but would then die from the drug's side-effects. More than half his survey said they would still take the drug.

[Performance-enhancing] drug users and their suppliers have become more skilled at evading [drug tests].

This seems to support other evidence that sport's problem with drugs is greater than it cares to admit. Indeed, of abuse in the past there is no longer any doubt. Secret police files uncovered in the former East Germany reveal a systematic and successful government-approved doping programme in the 1970s and 1980s to ensure that the communist regime could boast more sporting medals per head than its capitalist rivals.

What the East Germans were doing to their athletes, other communist block countries were surely doing too. So, too, were many western coaches. How else, ask the suspicious, could the human body—even with better diets, facilities and coaching methods—have improved so quickly its ability to run, jump, throw and swim?

Room for improvement

Have the 1990s, with the cold war over, seen a reduction in drug use? It is difficult to say. Judy Oakes, a British shot putter who is vehemently against drugs in sport, was ranked 27th in the world at her peak in 1988. By 1996, despite no improvement in her performance, she had climbed to 12th. The obvious conclusion is that she was no longer having to compete against so many drug-enhanced rivals. Michelle Verroken, head of the Ethics and Doping Directorate of the UK [United Kingdom] Sports Council, agrees that drug usage has probably declined. "If you're using drugs, you have to rely on a ring of silence," she argues. "Kiss and tell could be very attractive." She has a point: someone has to procure the drug for the naive young athlete and someone has to administer it in the right quantities. If drug use were rampant, surely the news would leak, or be sold, more frequently to a scandal-hungry media?

On the other hand, as recently as 1993, Belgium's Prince Alexandre de Merode, who is head of the International Olympic Committee's medical commission, said that he believed one-in-ten Olympic athletes was a regular drug user. Other experts claim that drug users are, in fact, a majority. Their answer to Mrs Verroken's argument is that to break the ring of silence around a drug user, even for a fat cheque from a newspaper, is to incriminate oneself—and then be shunned by official sporting bodies and sponsors. Meanwhile, there are plenty of sceptics who maintain that, although East Germany's abuse may have ended, China's is rampant.

At first their accusations were aimed at the Chinese women distance runners who dominated the 1993 World Championships in Germany. Could their spectacular success really have been achieved by hard work, caterpillar fungus and turtle blood, as their coach, Ma Junren, claimed? Increasingly the accusations are now being levelled against China's swimmers, who have climbed the world rankings during the 1990s while also being responsible for half the sport's positive tests since 1991. One Chinese swimmer, arriving for the world swimming championships in Australia in January, was found by customs to be carrying 13 vials of human growth hormone—turtle jelly, Chinese officials claimed—in her luggage. At the championships themselves, four Chinese swimmers tested positive for a banned diuretic (used to dilute urine samples so that anabolic steroids are not detected).

Are such results proof that the system is working, that top-level sport is becoming cleaner? It seems at least as likely that they merely reveal the tip of an iceberg.

One reason to join the sceptics is that, just as the testers have become more expert and intrusive—they now watch an athlete give his or her urine sample—so drug users and their suppliers have become more skilled at evading them. Water-based testosterone, for example, leaves the body in a day. A good drugs adviser will know exactly how much of a drug an athlete can take—and when he or she must stop. Andrew Jennings, a British journalist with little good to say about the management of athletics, points out that, before his fall from grace, Ben Johnson had passed 19 dope tests in two years.

A second reason for scepticism is that many of the testing parameters are so wide as to be almost meaningless. Because a few men and even fewer women have naturally high levels of testosterone, for example, the International Olympic Committee (IOC) has to adopt ratios which would not exclude them. The result is that most athletes could take regular doses of testosterone—thus boosting their performance, especially in the case of women athletes—without falling foul of the guidelines.

A third reason is that sports organisations feel legally vulnerable. Even the smallest mistake in the testing procedure could mean an expensive lawsuit from an athlete who sees his or her future earnings at risk. An American discus thrower once tested positive for the anabolic steroid, nandrolone—but he was exonerated because the doctor accidentally mislabelled one of the two sample bottles.

> *East German doping [performance-enhancing drug use] was very carefully regulated—and the results have been horrendous.*

Another American, Butch Reynolds, a 400-metres runner, tested positive for a steroid after a race in Monaco in 1990, and was banned for two years. Mr Reynolds steadfastly protested his innocence, alleged irregularities in the testing procedures and sought recourse against the International Amateur Athletics Federation in the American courts—which in 1992 awarded him $6.8m in lost earnings and $20.5m in punitive damages. The judgment was eventually set aside, but not before the sports world had collectively trembled at its implications.

There is one other reason to suspect an iceberg. Some doping methods simply cannot be satisfactorily detected by testing an athlete's urine (and for reasons, it says, of practicality and religious scruple the IOC has so far been reluctant to require blood-testing). Urine tests do not show human growth hormone, for example, nor added amounts of the cyclists' favourite, erythropoietin, a hormone that increases the formation of the red blood cells and so delivers more oxygen to the muscles.

The perils of permissiveness

Why not, then, abandon this definition of cheating as an exercise in futility? There is an intellectually respectable argument that goes as follows: sport is inherently unfair because contestants are born with different abilities, are trained by coaches with differing abilities and benefit from facilities of differing standards. The taking of drugs is just another way of gaining an advantage—and if it were legal, doping could be carefully monitored to ensure the sportsman comes to no harm.

Up to a point this argument, advanced by pragmatists and libertarians alike, is convincing enough. Sportsmen are clearly not all born equal or raised equally: a short Filipino, however obsessed with basketball, has no chance of slam-dunking with Michael Jordan and Shaquille O'Neal; a Jamaican brought up in the Caribbean will not win a downhill ski-race; American and European runners are beginning to feel they have no chance against distance runners from the Kenyan highlands who have spent their childhoods running several miles to school each day. As to the objection that rich countries have more chemists and better laboratories and so sportsmen from poor countries would suffer disproportionately from a doping free-for-all, surely pills, and the knowledge of how to use them, are a lot more transferable than the rich world's perfectly-groomed soccer pitches or Olympic-sized swimming pools.

But dig a little deeper and the argument shows its flaws. Would officially regulated doping really safeguard athletes? Given the pressure of competition, it seems inherently unlikely. In practice athletes would be guinea-pigs, taking drugs in doses well above any levels tested for safety by the manufacturers. East German doping was very carefully regulated—and the results have been horrendous: several male athletes have developed cancerous breasts. One depressing feature of the East German programme is that for many athletes the doping started in their childhood, when they could never have weighed the consequences.

And that is surely the greatest flaw in the argument. Professional sportsmen can be strange people, their values distorted by ambition, competition and money. But once upon a time they were just children, with innocent dreams of emulating their idealised heroes. If the heroes are seen to use drugs, then the hero-worshipping children will be tempted to do so as well.

That is something no sporting authority can afford. The reason is not just moral, compelling though that may be, but also commercial. The money for sport and its participants comes from television companies and sponsors; their money comes from attracting an audience that believes that sport should embody, to quote the Olympic charter, "a spirit of friendship, solidarity and fair play." That is why Ben Johnson lost his sponsors overnight and why—because of persistent rumours of drug use—

Ireland's Michelle Smith has failed to land the endorsement contracts she must surely have expected after winning three swimming gold medals at the Atlanta Olympics.

Cynics will say it is also why the Atlanta games were so "clean": it would have been commercially disastrous—for athletes, organisers, sponsors and broadcasters—to have them declared anything else.

6

Teen Steroid Abuse Is a Growing Problem

Steven Ungerleider

Steven Ungerleider is a clinical psychologist and an adjunct professor at the University of Oregon. He regularly consults with the U.S. Olympic Committee.

In response to social and athletic pressures to build greater strength and muscle, middle school and high school students are increasingly taking anabolic steroids. Steroids allow young athletes to train harder and recover more quickly from long workouts, but they pose numerous health risks to users. Side effects may include heart and liver damage and the premature cessation of bone growth in adolescents, which leads to shortened stature. More research is needed to address the dangerous consequences of adolescent steroid use.

In 1995, in a well-known research project, elite athletes were asked whether they would take a pill that guaranteed an Olympic gold medal if they knew it would kill them within a year. More than half of the athletes said they would take the pill.

The need to win at all costs has permeated many areas of our lives. In sports, one of the forms it takes is the use of anabolic-androgenic steroids (AAS). "Anabolic" refers to constructive metabolism or muscle-building, and "androgenic" means masculinizing. All AAS are derived from the hormone testosterone, which is found primarily in men, although women also produce it in smaller concentrations. There are at least thirty AAS, some natural and some synthetic.

A pervasive problem reaches young athletes

Use of these substances has been pervasive for years among collegiate, Olympic, and professional competitors. Experiments with steroids began in Germany in the thirties, and their use by East German Olympic athletes is well known. More than 10,000 East German athletes in 22 events were given these synthetic hormones over 30 years. In August 2000, after a long battle in the criminal courts, more than 400 doctors, coaches, and trainers from the former East Germany were convicted of giving steroids to minors without their informed consent. But despite these revelations and convictions, scandals persist. In June 2000, the chief of sports medicine for the United States Olympic Committee, Dr. Wade Exum, resigned in protest, saying that "some of our greatest Olympians have been using performance-enhancing drugs for years, and we have not been honest about our drug testing protocols."

Now anabolic steroids are becoming available to middle school and high school children as well. Concerns about body image and athletic performance lead adolescents to use the substances despite their serious side effects. Young athletes are responding to encouragement, social pressure, and their own desire to excel, as well as admonitions from coaches to put on muscle and build strength and resilience.

A recent survey by the National Institute on Drug Abuse indicates that steroid use by eighth- and tenth-graders is increasing, and twelfth-graders are increasingly likely to underestimate their risks. Some 2.7% of eighth- and tenth-graders and 2.9% of twelfth-graders admitted they had taken steroids at least once—a significant increase since 1991, the first year that full data were available. Other studies suggest that as many as 6% of high school students have used steroids. The numbers are espe-

Table 1: Side Effects of Anabolic-Androgenic Steroids

In men:
- Gynecomastia (breast development), usually permanent
- Testicular or scrotal pain
- Testicular atrophy and decreased sperm production
- Premature baldness, even in adolescents
- Enlargement of the prostate gland, causing difficult urination

In women:
- Enlargement of the clitoris, usually irreversible
- Disruption of the menstrual cycle
- Permanent deepening of the voice
- Excessive facial and body hair

In both sexes:
- Nervous tension
- Aggressiveness and antisocial behavior
- Paranoia and psychotic states
- Acne, often serious enough to leave permanent scars on the face and body
- Burning and pain during urination
- Gastrointestinal and leg muscle cramps
- Headaches
- Dizziness
- High blood pressure
- Heart, kidney, and liver damage
- In adolescents, premature end to the growth of long bones, leading to shortened stature

cially alarming because many students will not admit that they take drugs. Sixth-graders report that these drugs are available in schoolyards, and they are increasingly used by nonathletes as well to impress their peers and attract the opposite sex.

Anabolic-androgenic steroids fall into three classes: C-17 alkyl derivatives of testosterone; esters or derivatives of 19-nortestosterone; and esters of testosterone.

Concerns about body image and athletic performance lead adolescents to use [steroids] despite their serious side effects.

C-17 alkyl derivatives are soluble in water and can be taken orally. Among them are Anavar, Anadrol, Dianabol (a favorite among Olympians), and the most famous, Winstrol, also known as stanozolol. Stanozolol was taken in large doses by the Canadian sprint champion Ben Johnson, who was stripped of a gold medal in the 1988 Olympics. These steroids are often favored by athletes trying to avoid drug screens because they clear the body quickly (within a month).

The 19-nortestosterone derivatives are oil-based; they are usually injected and absorbed into fat deposits, where long-term energy is stored. The most popular steroid in this group is nandrolone (Deca-Durabolin). It has recently made headlines because it is found in food supplements and other preparations that can be bought without a prescription. Many athletes who test positive for nandrolone say they had no idea what was in the vitamin supplements they took. Because nandrolone is stored in fatty tissue and released over a long period of time, it may take 8–10 months to clear the body.

Esters of testosterone, the third class, are especially dangerous. Among them are testosterone propionate, Testex, and cypionate. Active both orally and by injection, they closely mimic the effects of natural testosterone and are therefore difficult to detect on drug screens. The International Olympic Committee determines their presence by measuring the ratio of testosterone to the related substance epitestosterone in an athlete's urine; if the ratio exceeds 6:1, the athlete is suspected of cheating.

Inducing irritability, aggression, and health risks

How do anabolic steroids work? The scientific literature demonstrates their effects, but it is not clear how they enhance the synthesis of proteins and the growth of muscles. They apparently increase endurance, allowing longer periods of exercise, and improve the results of strength training by increasing both the size (mass) of muscles and the number of muscle fibers.

Especially when taken in high doses, AAS can induce irritability and aggression. When Hitler's SS troops took steroids to build strength and stave off fatigue, they found that the hormones also made them more fearless and willing to fight. Among young athletic warriors today, steroids not only permit harder training and faster recovery from long workouts but may also induce a sense of invincibility and promote excessively macho behavior—and occasionally, attacks of rage or psychosis.

These drugs have a great many other risks as well. Men may develop reduced sperm production, shrunken testicles, impotence, and irreversible breast enlargement. Women may develop deep voices and excessive body hair. In either sex, baldness and acne are risks. The ratio of good to bad lipids may change, increasing the danger of heart attacks, strokes, and liver cancer. In adolescents bone growth may stop prematurely. (See Table 1 for details on side effects.) Injecting steroids with contaminated needles creates a risk of HIV and other blood-borne infections.

Mental health professionals must consider how to address this problem in our schools. The National Institute on Drug Abuse and its nongovernmental partners have established Web sites to educate youth about the dangers of steroids. These sites may be found at steroidabuse.org, archpediatrics.com, and drugabuse.gov. A useful site for professionals interested in intervention and prevention is tpronline.org. Researchers at the Oregon Health Sciences University have devised an effective program known as Adolescents Training and Learning to Avoid Steroids (ATLAS). It is a team-centered and gender-specific approach that educates athletes about the dangers of steroids and other drugs while providing alternatives including nutritional advice and strength training. A three-year study demonstrated the benefits of the program for 3,000 football players in 31 Oregon high schools. ATLAS reduced not only anabolic steroid use but also alcohol and illicit drug use and drunk driving. Still more research is needed both to address the potentially deadly consequences of youthful steroid use and to discover ways of preventing it.

7

Performance-Enhancing Drugs Compromise Medical Ethics

Philippe Liotard

Philippe Liotard is a professor at the Sports Faculty of the University of Monpellier, France, and the cofounder of Quasimodo *magazine.*

Medical ethics are being challenged by the demand for treatments intended to enhance a person's physical appearance and social performance, such as anti-aging treatments and cosmetic surgery, which are not directly related to the goal of good health. Doctors involved in sport medicine now find themselves at the center of this ethical dilemma. They face enormous pressure to go beyond merely treating an athlete's fatigue and pain to prescribing performance-enhancing drugs. However, doctors should not reinforce society's emphasis on performance at all costs by prescribing drugs that mask pain and illness and put an athlete's health in jeopardy.

On the eve of the Sydney Olympic Games [fall 2000], sport medicine is faced with ethical dilemmas that stretch well beyond the domain of top-level competition.

Advances in life sciences and biotechnology are stirring up a broad debate about ethics. Expert committees are being called upon to bring ethical codes in line with genetic research developments, assisted reproduction, prenatal screening and the prospects for human cloning.

Standards for clinical research on humans, spelt out in the 1947 Nuremberg Rules [following World War II], are now being challenged by medical advances and research unimaginable in those days. Questions surrounding the prospects of human embryo research (and the risks of new forms of eugenics) as well as research spurred by the mapping of the human genome, are generating new laws based on consultation with national and international ethics committees, along with medical and re-

From "Sport Medicine: To Heal or to Win?" by Philippe Liotard, *UNESCO Courier*, September 2000. Copyright © 2000 by UNESCO. Reprinted with permission.

search groups. This is the most public part of the debate, the issues that make headlines.

But medical ethics involve far more than these issues, which are all essential to imagining the kind of "humanity" that we are embarking to create. Tomorrow's society is being assembled day by day in the privacy of doctors' surgeries. For medical ethics are also being challenged by patients themselves, and by practices that have become routine.

A premium on efficiency and performance

Doctors are inevitably affected by societal changes, shifting aspirations and accepted behavioural norms. They also have to try, in their relationship with patients, to reconcile ethical considerations with the new demands arising from a liberal society that puts high value on efficiency, output and performance. This is especially true in the case of drug-taking (or doping) in sport, which can be seen as the logical outcome of a performance-based type of medical practice. Oddly enough, discussion about doping is generally reduced to a few cliches: it is branded as unethical in light of an imaginary sporting ideal. Calls are made for better drug-testing and stiffer punishment for "cheats" and their accomplices. But this skates over the real issue—the pressures of competition in sport— and hides it even further from the public, doctors and authorities.

Doping in high-pressure sports can hardly be equated with reckless or rash behaviour. On the contrary, it requires the conscious involvement of the competitor who personally controls the state of his or her own body and training. The athlete is led to take drugs daily to reduce fatigue and to increase muscle power, or to recover quickly from an injury or excessive training, for example. The scandal over the Tour de France bicycle race in 1998 showed how riders knowingly and personally take banned substances in order to endure tough training and back-to-back races throughout a whole season.

So the real ethical debate rests solely on medical practice. It means we should reflect on how doctors respond to requests from athletes at all levels, for doping is also on the rise among amateurs and children.

> *[Doctors must] reconcile ethical considerations with the new demands arising from a liberal society that puts high value on . . . performance.*

At the 43rd American Health Congress, held in Washington in September 1996, Thomas H. Murray, of the Center for Biomedical Ethics at Case Western Reserve University (Cleveland, Ohio), recounted how a mother asked for growth hormones for her son to improve his sporting performance. There are two factors behind this request. First, advances in medical biotechnology have made it possible to produce artificial hormones. Second, the drive to win draws the doctor into altering the body to make it perform better.

All medical codes of ethics condemn doctors acceding to such requests. The World Medical Association calls on every doctor to "oppose and refuse to administer or condone" methods that aim at "an unnatural increase or maintenance of performance during competition" or which "artificially change features appropriate to age and sex" (1981 Declaration on Principles of Health Care for Sport Medicine, amended in 1999).

Hormone boosts

But many doctors must still deal with the consequences of sporting activity. Physiologically, sport depletes a person's natural reserves, especially hormones. Intensive training for example, uses up the male hormone testosterone faster than the body replaces it. A doctor can put an athlete on supplements to make up for that loss, just as iron or vitamins are prescribed for people lacking them. So a deficiency in the body is made up for without any regard for what might have caused it in the first place—such as malnutrition, overwork or disease.

Doctors can still . . . refuse to play the game and deplore the effects of a hectic life-style imposed by the obligation to perform.

We do not yet have a separate branch of medicine dealing with performance. So far, it is just a few doctors straying from the original purposes of medicine. In the richest countries and among the elites in poor nations, such medicine is in demand as a medical prop to cope with the new emphasis placed on performance in all spheres of life. This is also very similar in principle to anti-ageing treatments, where health care is being adjusted to the fact that people are living longer. Hormone replacement therapy in elderly people is aimed at "improving the quality of life to match the extra number of years gained," according to Dr. Bruno Delignieres, head of the endocrinology service at the Necker Hospital in Paris. Here too, hormonal adjustment is being prescribed because of progress in life sciences and patients' requests for drugs to alleviate the effects of ageing. The doctor is responding to a person's natural desire to improve their physical condition. Just like cosmetic surgery and treatments for impotence, which have been boosted by the invention of the drug Viagra, medicine is turning towards satisfying desires, spurred by images of well-being and youth. The pressure to get, maintain or preserve an "efficient" body and a "slim" figure is steadily increasing. The same goes for reducing pain during childbirth, old age and of course in everyday life, which includes sporting activity.

So one might think there is nothing wrong with prescribing drugs which improve the quality of an athlete's life, marked by intense physical activity. Fighting against stress, recovering from long-term fatigue, using anti-inflammatory drugs to reduce pain caused by intense exertion become normal given social expectations of chemically-assisted well-being.

But testosterone and related products, such as nandrolone, are classified as anabolic steroids and are the substances most frequently detected during drug testing. When taken in big doses, together with sufficient food and training, testosterone increases body mass, strength and muscle power as well as aggressivity and resistance to fatigue and pain. Corticoid drugs also reduce pain and help a person to tire less easily. So these substances are very suitable for easing the physical effects and psychological pressures of competitive sport.

The crucial issue lies in deciding where medical efforts to restore equilibrium end and efforts to improve performance begin. An artificial dividing line has been drawn. A scale has been devised to measure the quantity of "supplements." Medical tests can now detect if a person has taken "unreasonable" amounts of substances that are no longer banned, but tolerated up to a certain point.

Medical ethics do not require a doctor to ask whether someone is "cheating" under the rules of sport. A doctor does not have to take a stand on demands made in fields other than his own. The problem is how to define the state of health that the doctor aims for, not the level of doping. The World Medical Association's Geneva Declaration (adopted in 1948 and amended in 1983) is clear: "The health of my patient will be my first consideration," a doctor is supposed to pledge. So it naturally condemns "procedures to mask pain or other protective symptoms if used to enable the athlete to take part in an event when lesions or signs are present which make his participation inadvisable."

Doctors (in sport or otherwise) who engage in these practices are not performing their duty towards patients (which involves prescribing a halt to painful activity) but are complying with the demands of sport. From an ethical standpoint, a desired performance must not be taken into account in the course of diagnosis or treatment. Medical ethics condemn any action dictated by interests or pressures not related to the goal of good health.

This is where the debate gets really tricky, because in modern parlance and in the language of doping in sport, good health is understood to mean the absence of illness or lasting after-effects. However, since 1940, the World Health Organization has defined good health as a combined state of physical, emotional and social well-being. The Centre for Health Promotion at the University of Toronto, points out that good health is not an end in itself but a means to a balanced life.

This makes good health a quest for well-being based on individual aspirations in a particular social and cultural context. Put this way, it becomes something extremely subjective and changeable according to the time and place as well as the sex, age and social class of the person involved. Each individual decides on the basis of his or her own life and cultural environment a relationship to well-being, pain and illness.

Sport presents doctors with a paradox. Most of them believe physical activity makes for a balanced life. But they are also well aware that competition upsets this balance, and that chemical-based treatments can be prescribed to supplement deficiencies. If they respond to such demands, they are only reinforcing the alienating emphasis put on performance at all costs, of which sport is just the most striking example.

Science at the altar of performance?

But doctors can still, without any qualms of conscience, refuse to play the game and deplore the effects of a hectic life-style imposed by the obligation to perform. Acting in the interest of patients' welfare involves teaching them how to pursue a balanced life. A doctor's duty is to tell patients why they are ill. If this can be done without problem where obesity and the dangers of smoking or drinking are concerned, the same goes where the dangerous effects of sport are involved.

Sport medicine is a forerunner of the medicine of the future—a medicine at the behest of institutions in the business of boosting efficiency. It runs the risk of ushering in a common norm dictating people's appearance (through cosmetic surgery), character (through prenatal diagnosis) and social behaviour, namely through the demand for performance in all fields, be it professional, sexual or sporting.

8

Performance-Enhancing Drugs Should Be Regulated, Not Prohibited

Malcolm Gladwell

Malcolm Gladwell is a staff writer for the New Yorker *magazine.*

Performance-enhancing drugs allow athletes to train harder and improve their athletic performance over a short period of time. Many of today's athletes take the drugs willingly and have grown increasingly uncertain about what is wrong with doing so. Drug testing by sports authorities is unreliable, and athletes are constantly taking new drugs for which no test has been devised. The attempt to ban certain drugs gives an advantage to those athletes with the means to take newer drugs. Instead of prohibiting performance-enhancing drugs, testing authorities should set acceptable limits for drug use. Regulating aggressive drug use will restore parity to sports, ensuring that no athlete can cheat more than another.

At the age of twelve, Christiane Knacke-Sommer was plucked from a small town in Saxony to train with the élite SC Dynamo swim club, in East Berlin. After two years of steady progress, she was given regular injections and daily doses of small baby-blue pills, which she was required to take in the presence of a trainer. Within weeks, her arms and shoulders began to thicken. She developed severe acne. Her pubic hair began to spread over her abdomen. Her libido soared out of control. Her voice turned gruff. And her performance in the pool began to improve dramatically, culminating in a bronze medal in the hundred-metre butterfly at the 1980 Moscow Olympics. But then the [Berlin] Wall fell and the truth emerged about those little blue pills. In a new book about the East German sports establishment, "Faust's Gold," Steven Ungerleider recounts the moment in 1998 when Knacke-Sommer testified in Berlin at the trial of her former coaches and doctors:

> "Did defendant Gläser or defendant Binus ever tell you that the blue pills were the anabolic steroid known as Oral-

From "Drugstore Athlete," by Malcolm Gladwell, *New Yorker*, September 10, 2001. Copyright © 2001 by the *New Yorker*. Reprinted with permission.

Turinabol?" the prosecutor asked. "They told us they were vitamin tablets," Christiane said, "just like they served all the girls with meals." "Did defendant Binus ever tell you the injection he gave was Depot-Turinabol?" "Never," Christiane said, staring at Binus until the slight, middle-aged man looked away. "He said the shots were another kind of vitamin."

"He never said he was injecting you with the male hormone testosterone?" the prosecutor persisted. "Neither he nor Herr Gläser ever mentioned Oral-Turinabol or Depot-Turinabol," Christiane said firmly. "Did you take these drugs voluntarily?" the prosecutor asked in a kindly tone. "I was fifteen years old when the pills started," she replied, beginning to lose her composure. "The training motto at the pool was, 'You eat the pills, or you die.' It was forbidden to refuse."

As her testimony ended, Knacke-Sommer pointed at the two defendants and shouted, "They destroyed my body and my mind!" Then she rose and threw her Olympic medal to the floor.

Anabolic steroids have been used to enhance athletic performance since the early sixties, when an American physician gave the drugs to three weight lifters, who promptly jumped from mediocrity to world records. But no one ever took the use of illegal drugs quite so far as the East Germans. In a military hospital outside the former East Berlin, in 1991, investigators discovered a ten-volume archive meticulously detailing every national athletic achievement from the mid-sixties to the fall of the Berlin Wall, each entry annotated with the name of the drug and the dosage given to the athlete. An average teen-age girl naturally produces somewhere around half a milligram of testosterone a day. The East German sports authorities routinely prescribed steroids to young adolescent girls in doses of up to thirty-five milligrams a day. As the investigation progressed, former female athletes, who still had masculinized physiques and voices, came forward with tales of deformed babies, inexplicable tumors, liver dysfunction, internal bleeding, and depression. German prosecutors handed down hundreds of indictments of former coaches, doctors, and sports officials, and won numerous convictions. It was the kind of spectacle that one would have thought would shock the sporting world. Yet it didn't. In a measure of how much the use of drugs in competitive sports has changed in the past quarter century, the trials caused barely a ripple.

Today, coaches no longer have to coerce athletes into taking drugs. Athletes take them willingly.

Today, coaches no longer have to coerce athletes into taking drugs. Athletes take them willingly. The drugs themselves are used in smaller doses and in creative combinations, leaving few telltale physical signs, and drug testers concede that it is virtually impossible to catch all the cheaters, or even, at times, to do much more than guess when cheating is taking place. Among the athletes, meanwhile, there is growing uncertainty about what exactly is wrong with doping. When the cyclist Lance Armstrong asserted last year [2000], after his second consecutive Tour de France victory, that he was drug-free, some doubters wondered whether he was lying, and others simply assumed he was, and wondered why he had to. The moral clarity of the East German scandal—with its coercive coaches, damaged athletes, and corrupted competitions—has given way to shades of gray. In today's climate, the most telling moment of the East German scandal was not Knacke-Sommer's outburst. It was when one of the system's former top officials, at the beginning of his trial, shrugged and quoted Brecht: "Competitive sport begins where healthy sport ends."

The quest for "quantum leaps"

Perhaps the best example of how murky the drug issue has become is the case of Ben Johnson, the Canadian sprinter who won the one hundred metres at the Seoul Olympics, in 1988. Johnson set a new world record, then failed a post-race drug test and was promptly stripped of his gold medal and suspended from international competition. No athlete of Johnson's calibre has ever been exposed so dramatically, but his disgrace was not quite the victory for clean competition that it appeared to be.

Among world-class athletes, the lure of steroids is . . . that they make it possible to train harder.

Johnson was part of a group of world-class sprinters based in Toronto in the nineteen-seventies and eighties and trained by a brilliant coach named Charlie Francis. Francis was driven and ambitious, eager to give his athletes the same opportunities as their competitors from the United States and Eastern Europe, and in 1979 he began discussing steroids with one of his prize sprinters, Angella Taylor. Francis felt that Taylor had the potential that year to run the two hundred metres in close to 22.90 seconds, a time that would put her within striking distance of the two best sprinters in the world, Evelyn Ashford, of the United States, and Marita Koch, of East Germany. But, seemingly out of nowhere, Ashford suddenly improved her two-hundred-metre time by six-tenths of a second. Then Koch ran what Francis calls, in his autobiography, "Speed Trap," a "science fictional" 21.71. In the sprints, individual improvements are usually measured in hundredths of a second; athletes, once they have reached their early twenties, typically improve their performance in small, steady increments, as experience and strength increase. But these were quantum leaps, and to Francis the explanation was obvious. "Angella wasn't losing ground because of a talent gap," he writes; "she was losing because of a drug gap, and it was widening by the day." (In the case of Koch, at least, he was right. In the East German archives, investigators found a letter from Koch to the director of research at V.E.B. Jenapharm, an East German pharmaceutical house, in which she complained, "My drugs were not as potent as the ones that were given to my opponent Bärbel Eckert, who kept beating me." In East Germany, Ungerleider writes, this particu-

ed by athletes to speed the metabolism and keep people lean." But the
anadians stuck to their initial regimen, making only a few changes: Vi-
min B$_{12}$, a non-steroidal muscle builder called inosine, and occasional
ots of testosterone were added; Dianabol was dropped in favor of a
ewer steroid called Furazabol; and L-dopa, which turned out to cause
iffness, was replaced with the blood-pressure drug Dixarit.

Unreliable testing

oing into the Seoul Olympics, then, Johnson was a walking pharmacy.
ut—and this is the great irony of his case—none of the drugs that were
art of his formal pharmaceutical protocol resulted in his failed drug test.
Ie had already reaped the benefit of the steroids in intense workouts lead-
ng up to the games, and had stopped Furazabol and testosterone long
nough in advance that all traces of both supplements should have disap-
eared from his system by the time of his race—a process he sped up by
aking the diuretic Moduret. Human growth hormone wasn't—and still
sn't—detectable by a drug test, and arginine, ornithine, and Dixarit were
egal. Johnson should have been clean. The most striking (and uninten-
ionally hilarious) moment in "Speed Trap" comes when Francis describes
his bewilderment at being informed that his star runner had failed a drug
test—for the anabolic steroid stanozolol. "I was floored," Francis writes:

> To my knowledge, Ben had never injected stanozolol. He
> occasionally used Winstrol, an oral version of the drug, but
> for no more than a few days at a time, since it tended to
> make him stiff. He'd always discontinued the tablets at least
> six weeks before a meet, well beyond the accepted "clear-
> ance time.". . . After seven years of using steroids, Ben knew
> what he was doing. It was inconceivable to me that he
> might take stanozolol on his own and jeopardize the most
> important race of his life.

Francis suggests that Johnson's urine sample might have been deliberately contaminated by a rival, a charge that is less preposterous than it
sounds. Documents from the East German archive show, for example,
that in international competitions security was so lax that urine samples
were sometimes switched, stolen from a "clean" athlete, or simply "bor-
rowed" from a noncompetitor. "The pure urine would either be infused
by a catheter into the competitor's bladder (a rather painful procedure) or
be held in condoms until it was time to give a specimen to the drug control lab," Ungerleider writes. (The top East German sports official Manfred
Höppner was once in charge of urine samples at an international weightlifting competition. When he realized that several of his weight lifters
would not pass the test, he broke open the seal of their specimens, poured
out the contents, and, Ungerleider notes, "took a nice long leak of pure
urine into them.") It is also possible that Johnson's test was simply
botched. Two years later, in 1990, track and field's governing body
claimed that Butch Reynolds, the world's four-hundred-metre record
holder, had tested positive for the steroid nandrolone, and suspended
him for two years. It did so despite the fact that half of his urine-sample
data had been misplaced, that the testing equipment had failed during

lar complaint was known as "dope-envy.") Later, Francis say:
fronted at a track meet by Brian Oldfield, then one of the
shot-putters:

> "When are you going to start getting serious?" h
> manded. "When are you going to tell your guys the fa
> life?" I asked him how he could tell they weren't alreac
> ing steroids. He replied that the muscle density just w
> there. "Your guys will never be able to compete agains
> Americans—their careers will be over," he persisted.

Training harder with drugs

Among world-class athletes, the lure of steroids is not that the)
transform performance—no drug can do that—but that they m
sible to train harder. An aging baseball star, for instance, may r
what he needs to hit a lot more home runs is to double the ir
his weight training. Ordinarily, this might actually hurt his per.
"When you're under that kind of physical stress," Charles Yesal
demiologist at Pennsylvania State University, says, "your bod
corticosteroids, and when your body starts making those hormo
appropriate times it blocks testosterone. And instead of being a
instead of building muscle—corticosteroids are catabolic. Th
down muscle. That's clearly something an athlete doesn't want.
steroids counteracts the impact of corticosteroids and helps t
bounce back faster. If that home-run hitter was taking testostero
anabolic steroid, he'd have a better chance of handling the extr
training.

---

*The basic problem with drug testing is that testers
are always one step behind athletes.*

It was this extra training that Francis and his sprinters fel
needed to reach the top. Angella Taylor was the first to start
steroids. Ben Johnson followed in 1981, when he was twenty yea
beginning with a daily dose of five milligrams of the steroid Dianal
three-week on-and-off cycles. Over time, that protocol grew more
plex. In 1984, Taylor visited a Los Angeles doctor, Robert Kerr, wh
famous for his willingness to provide athletes with pharmacologic
sistance. He suggested that the Canadians use human growth horn
the pituitary extract that promotes lean muscle and that had becom
Francis's words, "the rage in elite track circles." Kerr also recommer
three additional substances, all of which were believed to promote
body's production of growth hormone: the amino acids arginine anc
nithine and the dopamine precursor L-dopa. "I would later learn," F
cis writes, "that one group of American women was using three time
much growth hormone as Kerr had suggested, in addition to 15 i
ligrams per day of Dianabol, another 15 milligrams of Anavar, la
amounts of testosterone, and thyroxine, the synthetic thyroid horm(

analysis of the other half of his sample, and that the lab technician who did the test identified Sample H6 as positive—and Reynolds's sample was numbered H5. Reynolds lost the prime years of his career.

Regulating aggressive doping . . . is a better idea than trying to prohibit drug use.

We may never know what really happened with Johnson's assay, and perhaps it doesn't much matter. He *was* a doper. But clearly this was something less than a victory for drug enforcement. Here was a man using human growth hormone, Dixarit, inosine, testosterone, and Furazabol, and the only substance that the testers could find in him was stanozolol—which may have been the only illegal drug that he *hadn't* used. Nor is it encouraging that Johnson was the only prominent athlete caught for drug use in Seoul. It is hard to believe, for instance, that the sprinter Florence Griffith Joyner, the star of the Seoul games, was clean. Before 1988, her best times in the hundred metres and the two hundred metres were, respectively, 10.96 and 21.96. In 1988, a suddenly huskier FloJo ran 10.49 and 21.34, times that no runner since has even come close to equalling. In other words, at the age of twenty-eight—when most athletes are beginning their decline—Griffith Joyner transformed herself in one season from a career-long better-than-average sprinter to the fastest female sprinter in history. Of course, FloJo never failed a drug test. But what does that prove? FloJo went on to make a fortune as a corporate spokeswoman. Johnson's suspension cost him an estimated twenty-five million dollars in lost endorsements. The real lesson of the Seoul Olympics may simply have been that Johnson was a very unlucky man.

One step behind

The basic problem with drug testing is that testers are always one step behind athletes. It can take years for sports authorities to figure out what drugs athletes are using, and even longer to devise effective means of detecting them. Anabolic steroids weren't banned by the International Olympic Committee (I.O.C.) until 1975, almost a decade after the East Germans started using them. In 1996, at the Atlanta Olympics, five athletes tested positive for what we now know to be the drug Bromantan, but they weren't suspended, because no one knew at the time what Bromantan was. (It turned out to be a Russian-made psycho-stimulant.) Human growth hormone, meanwhile, has been around for twenty years, and testers still haven't figured out how to detect it.

Perhaps the best example of the difficulties of drug testing is testosterone. It has been used by athletes to enhance performance since the fifties, and the International Olympic Committee announced that it would crack down on testosterone supplements in the early nineteen-eighties. This didn't mean that the I.O.C. was going to test for testosterone directly, though, because the testosterone that athletes were getting from a needle or a pill was largely indistinguishable from the testosterone they produce naturally. What was proposed, instead, was to compare the level of testosterone in urine with the level of another hormone, epitestosterone, to determine what's called the T/E ratio. For most people, under normal circumstances, that ratio is 1:1, and so the theory was that if testers found a lot more testosterone than epitestosterone it would be a sign that the athlete was cheating. Since a small number of people have naturally high levels of testosterone, the I.O.C. avoided the risk of falsely accusing anyone by setting the legal limit at 6:1.

Did this stop testosterone use? Not at all. Through much of the eighties and nineties, most sports organizations conducted their drug testing only at major competitions. Athletes taking testosterone would simply do what Johnson did, and taper off their use in the days or weeks prior to those events. So sports authorities began randomly showing up at athletes' houses or training sites and demanding urine samples. To this, dopers responded by taking extra doses of epitestosterone with their testosterone, so their T/E would remain in balance. Testers, in turn, began treating elevated epitestosterone levels as suspicious, too. But that still left athletes with the claim that they were among the few with naturally elevated testosterone. Testers, then, were forced to take multiple urine samples, measuring an athlete's T/E ratio over several weeks. Someone with a naturally elevated T/E ratio will have fairly consistent ratios from week to week. Someone who is doping will have telltale spikes—times immediately after taking shots or pills when the level of the hormone in his blood soars. Did all these precautions mean that cheating stopped? Of course not. Athletes have now switched from injection to transdermal testosterone patches, which administer a continuous low-level dose of the hormone, smoothing over the old, incriminating spikes. The patch has another advantage: once you take it off, your testosterone level will drop rapidly, returning to normal, depending on the dose and the person, in as little as an hour. "It's the peaks that get you caught," says Don Catlin, who runs the U.C.L.A. [University of California at Los Angeles] Olympic Analytical Laboratory. "If you took a pill this morning and an unannounced test comes this afternoon, you'd better have a bottle of epitestosterone handy. But, if you are on the patch and you know your own pharmacokinetics, all you have to do is pull it off." In other words, if you know how long it takes for you to get back under the legal limit and successfully stall the test for that period, you can probably pass the test. And if you don't want to take that chance, you can just keep your testosterone below 6:1, which, by the way, still provides a whopping performance benefit. "The bottom line is that only careless and stupid people ever get caught in drug tests," Charles Yesalis says. "The elite athletes can hire top medical and scientific people to make sure nothing bad happens, and you can't catch them."

Regulation over prohibition

But here is where the doping issue starts to get complicated, for there's a case to be made that what looks like failure really isn't—that regulating aggressive doping, the way the 6:1 standard does, is a better idea than trying to prohibit drug use. Take the example of erythropoietin, or EPO. EPO is a hormone released by your kidneys that stimulates the production of red blood cells, the body's oxygen carriers. A man-made version of the hormone is given to those with suppressed red-blood-cell counts, like patients undergoing kidney dialysis or chemotherapy. But over the past decade it has also become the drug of choice for endurance athletes, because its ability to increase the amount of oxygen that the blood can carry to the muscles has the effect of postponing fatigue. "The studies that have attempted to estimate EPO's importance say it's worth about a three-, four-, or five-per-cent advantage, which is huge," Catlin says. EPO also has the advantage of being a copy of a naturally occurring substance, so it's very hard to tell if someone has been injecting it. (A cynic would say that this had something to do with the spate of remarkable times in endurance races during that period.)

So how should we test for EPO? One approach, which was used in the late nineties by the International Cycling Union, is a test much like the T/E ratio for testosterone. The percentage of your total blood volume which is taken up by red blood cells is known as your hematocrit. The average adult male has a hematocrit of between thirty-eight and forty-four per cent. Since 1995, the cycling authorities have declared that any rider who had a hematocrit above fifty per cent would be suspended—a deliberately generous standard (like the T/E ratio) meant to avoid falsely accusing someone with a naturally high hematocrit. The hematocrit rule also had the benefit of protecting athletes' health. If you take too much EPO, the profusion of red blood cells makes the blood sluggish and heavy, placing enormous stress on the heart. In the late eighties, at least fifteen professional cyclists died from suspected EPO overdoses. A fifty-per-cent hematocrit limit is below the point at which EPO becomes dangerous.

Even as we assert this distinction [between natural advantages and drug use] on the playing field . . . we defy it in our own lives.

But, like the T/E standard, the hematocrit standard had a perverse effect: it set the legal limit so high that it actually encouraged cyclists to titrate their drug use up to the legal limit. After all, if you are riding for three weeks through the mountains of France and Spain, there's a big difference between a hematocrit of forty-four per cent and one of 49.9 per cent. This is why Lance Armstrong faced so many hostile questions about EPO from the European press—and why eyebrows were raised at his five-year relationship with an Italian doctor who was thought to be an expert on performance-enhancing drugs. If Armstrong had, say, a hematocrit of forty-four per cent, the thinking went, why *wouldn't* he have raised it to 49.9, particularly since the rules (at least, in 2000) implicitly allowed him to do so. And, if he didn't, how on earth did he win?

The problems with hematocrit testing have inspired a second strategy, which was used on a limited basis at the Sydney Olympics and this summer's World Track and Field Championships. This test measures a number of physiological markers of EPO use, including the presence of reticulocytes, which are the immature red blood cells produced in large numbers by EPO injections. If you have a lot more reticulocytes than normal, then there's a good chance you've used EPO recently. The blood work is followed by a confirmatory urinalysis. The test has its weaknesses. It's really only useful in picking up EPO used in the previous week or so, whereas the benefits of taking the substance persist for a month. But there's no question that, if random EPO testing were done aggressively in the weeks leading to a major competition, it would substantially reduce cheating.

Limits allow parity

On paper, this second strategy sounds like a better system. But there's a perverse effect here as well. By discouraging EPO use, the test is simply pushing savvy athletes toward synthetic compounds called hemoglobin-based oxygen carriers, which serve much the same purpose as EPO but for which there is no test at the moment. "I recently read off a list of these new blood-oxygen expanders to a group of toxicologists, and none had heard of any of them," Yesalis says. "That's how fast things are moving." The attempt to prevent EPO use actually promotes inequity: it gives an enormous advantage to those athletes with the means to keep up with the next wave of pharmacology. By contrast, the hematocrit limit, though more permissive, creates a kind of pharmaceutical parity. The same is true of the T/E limit. At the 1986 world swimming championships, the East German Kristin Otto set a world record in the hundred-metre freestyle, with an extraordinary display of power in the final leg of the race. According to East German records, on the day of her race Otto had a T/E ratio of 18:1. Testing can prevent that kind of aggressive doping; it can insure no one goes above 6:1. That is a less than perfect outcome, of course, but international sports is not a perfect world. It is a place where Ben Johnson is disgraced and FloJo runs free, where Butch Reynolds is barred for two years and East German coaches pee into cups—and where athletes without access to the cutting edge of medicine are condemned to second place. Since drug testers cannot protect the purity of sport, the very least they can do is to make sure that no athlete can cheat more than any other.

Running on more than natural ability

The first man to break the four-minute mile was the Englishman Roger Bannister, on a windswept cinder track at Oxford, nearly fifty years ago. Bannister is in his early seventies now, and one day last summer he returned to the site of his historic race along with the current world-record holder in the mile, Morocco's Hicham El Guerrouj. The two men chatted and compared notes and posed for photographs. "I feel as if I am looking at my mirror image," Bannister said, indicating El Guerrouj's similarly tall, high-waisted frame. It was a polite gesture, an attempt to suggest that he and El Guerrouj were part of the same athletic lineage. But, as both men surely knew, nothing could be further from the truth.

Bannister was a medical student when he broke the four-minute mile in 1954. He did not have time to train every day, and when he did he squeezed in his running on his hour-long midday break at the hospital. He had no coach or trainer or entourage, only a group of running partners who called themselves "the Paddington lunch time club." In a typical workout, they might run ten consecutive quarter miles—ten laps—

with perhaps two minutes of recovery between each repetition, then gobble down lunch and hurry back to work. Today, that training session would be considered barely adequate for a high-school miler. A month or so before his historic mile, Bannister took a few days off to go hiking in Scotland. Five days before he broke the four-minute barrier, he stopped running entirely, in order to rest. The day before the race, he slipped and fell on his hip while working in the hospital. Then he ran the most famous race in the history of track and field. Bannister was what runners admiringly call an "animal," a natural.

El Guerrouj, by contrast, trains five hours a day, in two two-and-a-half-hour sessions. He probably has a team of half a dozen people working with him: at the very least, a masseur, a doctor, a coach, an agent, and a nutritionist. He is not in medical school. He does not go hiking in rocky terrain before major track meets. When Bannister told him, last summer, how he had prepared for his four-minute mile, El Guerrouj was stunned. "For me, a rest day is perhaps when I train in the morning and spend the afternoon at the cinema," he said. El Guerrouj certainly has more than his share of natural ability, but his achievements are a reflection of much more than that: of the fact that he is better coached and better prepared than his opponents, that he trains harder and more intelligently, that he has found a way to stay injury free, and that he can recover so quickly from one day of five-hour workouts that he can follow it, the next day, with another five-hour workout.

Steroids versus honest effort

Of these two paradigms, we have always been much more comfortable with the first: we want the relation between talent and achievement to be transparent, and we worry about the way ability is now so aggressively managed and augmented. Steroids bother us because they violate the honesty of effort: they permit an athlete to train too hard, beyond what seems reasonable. EPO fails the same test. For years, athletes underwent high-altitude training sessions, which had the same effect as EPO—promoting the manufacture of additional red blood cells. This was considered acceptable, while EPO is not, because we like to distinguish between those advantages which are natural or earned and those which come out of a vial.

Even as we assert this distinction on the playing field, though, we defy it in our own lives. We have come to prefer a world where the distractable take Ritalin, the depressed take Prozac, and the unattractive get cosmetic surgery to a world ruled, arbitrarily, by those fortunate few who were born focussed, happy, and beautiful. Cosmetic surgery is not "earned" beauty, but then natural beauty isn't earned, either. One of the principal contributions of the late twentieth century was the moral deregulation of social competition—the insistence that advantages derived from artificial and extraordinary intervention are no less legitimate than the advantages of nature. All that athletes want, for better or worse, is the chance to play by those same rules.

9

Ban Athletes Who Don't Use Steroids

Sidney Gendin

Sidney Gendin is the author of More Steroids, Please, *and is a retired professor of philosophy from Eastern Michigan University.*

Governments and sports federations are wrong for continuing to ban the use of performance-enhancing drugs like steroids. Steroids are less hazardous to human health than smoking or drinking, and society has traditionally permitted people to engage in risky activities, such as mountain climbing, when the danger posed only affects the individual involved. In addition, ineffective and more costly dietary supplements, which falsely claim to work just like steroids, are legal. Steroid use by athletes should not be considered unnatural or cheating—the drugs simply allow athletes to perform at their very best.

Isn't it time for the brainwashed public to know the truth about steroids? In their ideological zeal to ban "performance enhancing" drugs, national governments and the various local and international sports federations have ignorantly and self-righteously declared that steroid use is cheating, dangerous, and stupid. In fact, in general, it is neither dangerous nor stupid and it is cheating only because it has been capriciously commanded to be so.

Steroid dangers are minimal

In the first place, with respect to the alleged danger, people ought to know that there are dozens of steroids and it would be absurd to imagine that their risks are identical. Moreover, steroids come in two broad classes—the orals and the injectables. It is true that most of the orals have associated hazards but not a single one of them is as hazardous as smoking or drinking. The principle dangers of the injectables result from overdosing and, even so, they are mainly such alarming matters as acne and severe headache. Every legally obtainable prescription drug comes with a warning of dozens of worse side effects.

But what is that to you and me? Why should we legislate what risks people should run unless they can interfere with the rest of us? In our democratic, capitalist society many persons risk their last few dollars to start up businesses which will probably fail. We do not stop them. If and when they become multimillionaires we congratulate them. We don't permit people to drive without seatbelts because their accidents drive up insurance rates for the rest of us but we let people engage in the far riskier business of climbing mountains since the danger is mainly self-regarding. So enough virtue-parading preaching.

Product hypocrisy

As for the so-called cheating, who really are the cheaters? The average steroid user spends about $100–150 per month while the supplement industries grow rich on suckering in the hundreds of thousands, possibly millions, of foolish people spending up to $1000 per month on a variety of mumbo jumbo: androstenedione, 4-androstenedione, 19-androstenedione, androstenediol and the several 4, 5, 17, and 19 varieties of androstenediol, tribulus terrestris, enzymatic conversion accelerators, growth hormone stimulators, hormone-releasing peptides, testosterone "boosters," dozens of magical herbs and a ridiculous number of "non drugs" with unpronounceable names so they are always abbreviated such as HMB and DHEA. On top of all this, these folks who tend to be more affluent than steroid users, are pumping protein powders into their milk—$9 per day—and gobbling down protein candy bars—up to $3 each—while saving a bit of energy for screaming "Foul! Cheater!" at the poor steroid user. They are told by the manufacturers and distributors of these outlandish products that they look like steroids, feel like steroids and work like steroids. So? Why not ban them like steroids?

Not a single [orally administered steroid] is as hazardous as smoking or drinking.

But I say ban them and only them. For one thing, they don't work as well as steroids. More importantly, what care I as a fan that someone sets a remarkable record because he used steroids? I pay money to see sporting events and I am entitled to an athlete's very best. Isaac Stern can afford a violin that few violinists and no high school orchestra player can afford. Is he taking unfair advantage of them? If I pay $60 to hear Stern and learn his tone was not up to par because he was too lazy to bring his own violin and borrowed a $50 one from a high school kid, I justifiably want my money back. What care I that he usually plays upon a $200,000 instrument? I am not bothered by this; I want his very best. Likewise, I want the very best an athlete can give me. I don't want to watch athletes who could have done better if only they had used steroids. Talk of steroid performance as unnatural is as ridiculous as complaining about artificial hearts. As for me I plan to have a T-shirt made for me that will read on its front: "Use steroids or go home. Enough of crying and whining."

10

Coming Soon: Open Olympics!

Oliver Morton

Oliver Morton is a freelance writer and a contributing editor at Wired *and* Newsweek International.

The use of performance-enhancing drugs should be permitted in an Open Olympics that would take place alongside a separate Olympics in which drug use is prohibited. Instead of feeling compelled to take drugs in order to compete effectively, athletes would have a real choice as to whether or not they will remain drug-free. This parallel system would also offer greater protection to the health and well-being of those athletes who decide to use drugs, since they could openly seek the advice of health professionals. Using drugs to boost performance is just another manifestation of the way people have blurred the boundary between the human and the technological.

The Tour de France has a glorious history—think of Eddy Merckx's winning all three jerseys in 1969, Louison Bobet's heyday in the 1950s, the epic 1910 battle between Francois Faber and Octave Lapize. But as this year's prologue gets underway at Puy du Fou on July 3, there will be just one previous race on most people's minds—last year's, when the discovery of systematic doping in the top-ranking Festina team and elsewhere plunged the event into chaos. There were arrests, expulsions and go-slows [protests staged by riders] (a case of Festina exeunt, omnes lentes); only 88 of 189 competitors completed the competition.

As Graeme Fife's thorough and engaging recent book "Tour de France" makes clear, the Tour is an exceptional event (in what other sport is the United States represented by its postal service?). In drug use, though, it is simply at one end of a spectrum. Cyclists—competitors in the only motor sport where the driver is the motor—probably take drugs more routinely than other athletes and have been at it for longer. Some relied on strychnine-and-speed-ball boosts to get through the 19th century's hellish six-day endurance races. But the difference is one of degree, not of kind.

The sporting establishment decries drugs as the product of an unsportsmanlike win-at-all-costs mentality. It then says that it must, at all costs, win the war on drugs. When this accepted truth is challenged, two justifications are offered. One is the protection of athletes, particularly young ones, who worry that they will have to use drugs in order to compete. Second, it is said that to use a drug is to be untrue to the ideal of what an athlete should be. Both of these objections are understandable, especially the first. But neither is an argument against the open use of drugs in sport, as long as events for the undrugged take place in parallel. An honorable division of the spoils could end the war for good, by giving fair opportunities for victory both to those who take drugs and to those who don't.

Fair opportunities for [Olympic] victory [should be given] both to those who take drugs and to those who don't.

Imagine two Olympics: Olympics Classic, without drugs and with stringent random blood tests and lifetime bans to keep it that way; the Open Olympics, with pharmaceutical enhancements of all kinds openly reported, medically monitored, perhaps sponsored by drug companies. In the first you find athletes who believe that, while high-tech equipment is fine, high-tech drugs and scientifically augmented metabolisms aren't. In the second you find those who have made the decision that citius, altius, fortius [the Olympic motto—faster, higher, stronger] requires whatever it takes.

Some will argue that the Open Olympians would be putting themselves at risk. After all, a number of young cyclists have died in the past decade and circumstances suggest that drugs—notably the blood-thickener EPO—were to blame; the tell-all memoir by Willy Voet, the Festina team's soigneur, whose arrest with a car full of dope set off last year's fiasco, is called "Massacre a la chaine"—serial murder. But it is the unsupervised use of unsuitable drugs and of regimes designed to disguise that use from the authorities that are deadly. The Festina team's approach of systematic and supervised drug enhancement, though it broke the rules, at least tried to ensure a certain amount of safety for the cyclists.

"Vous etes tous des assassins!" [you are all assassins] screamed Lapize as he reached the top of the Tour's first-ever Pyrenean stage; he was shouting at the race's marshals, not its drug peddlers. On something as grueling as the Tour, athletes risk their health, whether they take drugs or not. Sporting accidents of all sorts regularly cripple and kill both adults and children the world over. Drugs taken voluntarily, openly and with professional advice will add to these risks far less than they do when taken in a culture of hearsay and secrecy. The need to hide drug taking is currently a significant added risk to the cheats who indulge. And openness builds much-needed expertise. In an Open Olympics, especially one in which pharmaceutical companies were involved as sponsors, there would be a strong incentive for effective but comparatively safe dosing regimes to be found and promulgated. Ways might be found to make drugged sports safer than undrugged ones—and in the long run, such knowledge could help the nonathletic masses.

Those masses, after all, are no strangers to drugs and their effects. And as scientific understanding of the body's workings grows, and as pharmaceutical companies find new products and strategies for appealing to the healthy—a larger if less motivated market than the sick—drugs of enhancement will reach into more and more lives. The tricky trade-offs between the benefits a treatment might bring and the tolls it might exact will become decisions faced by all. Athletes who refuse drugs may eventually come to be seen as quaint anachronisms, a touch perverse even if oddly admirable—rather in the way that vegetarians were a few decades ago, or those who champion vinyl over CDs are today.

People have long since moved beyond a state of nature in the ways in which they make things, go places, reproduce themselves and spend Saturday nights. In the next century our bodies will move farther and farther from the imperfect state in which evolution left them before being interrupted by medicine. The boundary between the human and the technological will become increasingly blurred. In this the man-machine symbiosis of competitive cycling, the quintessential cyborg sport, shows the way. The technological redefinition of the human will be the cultural main event of the coming century. By showing that what we value in the human spirit can survive this new symbiosis, sport can play a vital part in it. But only if the drugged and the undrugged are treated equally.

11

The Health Risks of Steroid Use Have Been Exaggerated

Rick Collins

Rick Collins is a bodybuilder and criminal defense attorney in New York state who has defended dozens of clients involved with the use and sale of anabolic steroid products.

The medical establishment's characterization of steroids as dangerous is a scare tactic promulgated to preserve the "purity" of athletic competition. Past studies concluding that steroids are ineffective at promoting muscle growth and cause irreversible side effects are not credible and were based on faulty methodology. While there are health risks associated with steroid use, particularly for women and adolescents, recent research indicates that adverse side effects, such as liver damage and psychiatric problems, have been highly overstated. Forty years of steroid use by athletes provides no evidence of a serious health crisis or epidemic of steroid-related deaths. Congress should reconsider its ban on the non-medical use of steroids by athletes.

While the primary objective of Congress in classifying anabolic steroids as controlled substances (and criminalizing their use) was probably to solve the pharmacologic "cheating" problem in competition sports, the reported health risks associated with these "deadly drugs" provided a seemingly valid basis for the legislation. The reportedly devastating health hazards were used to justify a policy favoring imprisonment of athletes involved with steroids over allowing them to "destroy themselves" with these substances. But would such a policy be appropriate if the real health dangers to healthy adult males were actually significantly less than the members of Congress—and the general public—have been led to believe? An unbiased review of the medical and scientific evidence of risks to healthy adult males is necessary in order to understand and assess the legitimacy of our current national approach to the "steroid problem."

Medical hyperbole

Regrettably, the medical and scientific community has historically been less than truthful in presenting information about anabolic steroids to the general public. For example, for many years their position was that steroids do not build muscle. . . . Even as late as 1984, in the highly publicized anti-steroid book *Death in the Locker Room: Steroids & Sports*, then-medical student Bob Goldman seriously presented his theory about how steroids work in a subchapter devoted to the "placebo effect." It is unclear whether such faulty opinions were based upon ignorance of the overwhelming anecdotal evidence or upon an attempt to protect the public by concealing the truth. Whatever the reason, "[t]he medical community lost much credibility as a result of repeated denials that [steroids] enhance performance," [according to Charles Yesalis and Virginia Cowart in *The Steroids Game*]. Of course, the athletes themselves knew decades earlier about the dramatic effects of anabolics on sports performance and appearance. While today the medical establishment concedes that there is no doubt that anabolic steroids do indeed work (perhaps too well), its previous position created a tremendous distrust within the athletic community and led to an often recognized polarization between the groups which may never be undone.

Athletes are convinced that doctors and the government advance the "side effect" argument mostly as a scare tactic.

Regarding anabolic steroid side effects and health hazards, the position of the medical community has been mostly linked to hyperbolic, hysterical works like *Death in the Locker Room*. The mainstream media, always seeking the sensationalism of a "big story," conveyed such material to the public as if it were gospel truth. With no personal experience to the contrary, the average American accepts this characterization of steroids as dangerous killer drugs. On the other hand, many strength athletes are convinced that doctors and the government advance the "side effect" argument mostly as a scare tactic to preserve the "purity" of athletic competition. They have amassed their own body of underground anecdotal evidence derived from their observations of side effects on themselves and on their peers, or from "underground" treatises on self-administration of steroids. "Athletes using anabolic steroids today have a sophisticated pharmacologic knowledge base for using these agents that surpasses that of the vast majority of physicians. For this reason, traditional warnings regarding the lack of efficacy and the potential dangers of steroid abuse are universally held in contempt. Today, it appears that the experts on anabolic steroid use in athletic competition are not medical clinicians but the athletes [themselves]," [according to researcher P.J. Perry].

Unreliable anabolic steroid research

Several problems have affected much of the past research into anabolic steroid effects. Until very recently, it was considered unethical for researchers to administer the highly supraphysiologic dosages necessary to simulate use patterns of established steroid users. Therefore, most human studies involved steroid users self-reporting their histories of dosages and duration of use, rather than any controlled administration by the researchers. The reliability problems with this methodology have been noted by experts in the field. Only recently have researchers begun to administer more substantial dosages for short-term periods, simulating the moderate-dose steroid cycles used by some athletes.

No case of permanent sterility as a result of prolonged high-dose steroid consumption has ever been reliably documented.

Another problem plaguing steroid research has been lack of funding. However, the growing interest in anabolic steroids for anti-aging and AIDS therapies may prompt grants for further research. Perhaps the most enlightening research would be retrospective cohort studies examining the health condition, cancer prevalence and mortality statistics of professional bodybuilders from the 1950's, 1960's and 1970's. With such studies, the long-term health ramifications of steroid use finally would be known and quantified. Regrettably, grant proposals to conduct such studies have been repeatedly turned down. Of course, a finding that there are generally no statistically significant long-term adverse effects (especially with moderate dosages and intermittent use) could encourage or increase non-medical steroid use, and might call into question our present national policy of criminalizing steroid users. Consequently, it is unlikely that a strong anti-steroid authority like the National Institute on Drug Abuse, a frequent sponsor of steroid research, will ever approve or fund such a study.

Anabolic steroid use by women and teenagers

Without question, there are health risks involved in the self-administration of any prescription medicine, particularly in the absence of a physician's advice with respect to dosages and duration of use. Further, without regular monitoring by a doctor, some side effects may go unnoticed or untreated until it is too late. Anabolic steroids can have adverse effects upon the body, and the risks for teenagers and women are higher than for adult males. Since large exogenous doses of androgens are more foreign to a woman's body than to a man's, their effect on the delicate hormonal balance of a woman is more profound. Excessive growth of body hair (hirsutism), coarsening of the skin, male pattern baldness, and deepening of the voice may occur (especially at massive dosages) and are generally not reversible upon discontinuance of steroids. Other possible effects particular to women include heavy facial masculinization, breast tissue reduction, alterations in menstrual cycles, and clitoral enlargement. Legal issues aside, any woman considering the use of high-dose androgens for physical enhancement must seriously weigh the perceived benefits against the quite unappealing potential cosmetic costs.

For teenagers, there is the additional risk of premature closure of the growth plates of the long bones. Even if not for this added risk, the self-administration of anabolics by teenagers must be strongly discouraged. As compared to mature adults, teenagers are much more likely to abuse anabolic steroids to the possible detriment of their health. Generally less focused upon long-range health than adults, more susceptible to peer pressure, and eager for fast results, teenagers are more likely to use anabolics in dangerously high dosages and without any medical supervision. Also, as it is recognized that the effects of anabolics upon size and strength are partially (and sometimes even completely) temporary, teens seem particularly less willing to suffer these post-cycle size and strength reductions, and are more likely to continuously use high-dose steroids for prolonged periods. Even Dan Duchaine, author of the *Underground Steroid Handbook II* and a favorite target of the proponents of steroid criminalization, is opposed to steroid use by teenagers. Clearly, even in countries where steroids can be legally obtained without a prescription, it is this writer's opinion that the choice to use them for physical enhancement should be made by mature, informed adults with a pre-established dedication to serious weight-training for several years. Anabolic steroids should never be used by beginning lifters, those with dubious commitments to weight-training, or those simply seeking a substitute for hard work. . . .

Adverse effects of excess androgens

The average adult male production of testosterone is less than 10 milligrams (mg) per day. Supplemental androgens can raise blood androgen levels to many times the amount that could be naturally produced. All these extra androgens will effect the body's hormonal balance, including the reproductive system. Because anabolics mimic endogenous androgens (i.e., your own natural testosterone) in the negative feedback loop of the hypothalamic-pituitary-gonadal axis, they cause the body to decrease its own production. Exactly how long it takes for the body to begin to shut down its own production of androgens is uncertain, although some have estimated it at about three weeks of steroid therapy. This induced hypogonadal state is characterized by decreased serum testosterone levels, associated testicular atrophy, and impaired sperm production that results in temporary infertility. It is this aspect of anabolic therapy that has been the focus of numerous studies testing the use of anabolics as a form of male contraception. But it is important to note that these effects are reversible with discontinuance of the steroids, and that no case of permanent sterility as a result of prolonged high-dose steroid consumption has ever been reliably documented.

> *Recent studies continue to suggest that reports of serious adverse effects of anabolic steroids . . . may be highly overstated.*

Steroid use can also effect the libido. It is common for the sex drive to heighten during a cycle but decrease toward the end and after because the body's own production of testosterone has been temporarily shut down due to the exogenous steroids. Decreased testicular size is also not uncommon with prolonged usage. Both of these adverse effects are reversible upon the body's own recuperation and often can be avoided altogether with the administration of gonadotropin stimulating drugs, which "jump-start" the body's natural production of testosterone.

"High dose equals high risk, . . . [but] low-dose [steroids] . . . pose little threat to health."

Other adverse effects of excessive androgens upon the body's system of hormones are primarily due to the eventual conversion of the androgens into other compounds. Steroid molecules in the body are eventually converted into other compounds or excreted in the urine. Testosterone can be converted by an enzymatic process into a slightly altered derivative hormone called dihydrotestosterone (DHT), a steroid molecule that may be significantly responsible for these adverse effects. Adverse effects of an androgenic nature occur because muscles are not the only parts of the body with receptor sites for steroid molecules, and because a steroid molecule has the potential to deliver several different messages. Which message the steroid molecule delivers depends upon the location of the receptor site to which it links. A steroid molecule linking to a receptor site in a hair follicle may deliver a message to stop growing (leading to male pattern baldness). One linking to a site in a sebaceous gland may deliver a message to produce more oil (leading to acne). One linking to a site in the prostate gland may deliver a message for the gland to enlarge (leading to prostatitis). The occurrence and extent of these adverse effects depend upon the concentration of receptor sites for steroid molecules in that particular area. Each individual is different. For example, male pattern baldness can be exacerbated in athletes who have a genetic predisposition. Steroids with a high conversion rate to DHT seem to be particularly responsible for this adverse effect, and should be avoided. Also, the effect can be partially controlled by the use of finasteride (Proscar or Propecia), a prescription drug which helps to block the conversion of testosterone to DHT.

The appearance of androgenic effects is also largely related to the dosage and to the choice of steroid. Highly androgenic steroids such as testosterone esters, especially in very large doses, will generally be much more prone to cause problems than highly anabolic, less androgenic drugs like methenolone or oxandrolone. However, recent research suggests that the side effects of even highly androgenic compounds have been overstated. There were no significant side effects of 10 weeks of testosterone enanthate at a dosage of 600 mg per week (six times the replacement dose of this highly androgenic ester and more than many bodybuilders might use). (In a discouraging kick in the pants to natural athletes everywhere, study participants receiving the testosterone injections without any exercise at all enjoyed significantly greater increases in fat-free mass, arm size and leg size than those who worked out hard but without the steroids.) Other studies have also reported minimal signifi-

cant androgenic side effects, including one involving the highly androgenic oral steroid oxymetholone. Androgens also have the capacity to be
converted into estrogen by chemical reactions and enzymes within certain body tissues. The process by which the steroid molecule is converted
to estrogen is called aromatization. Those anabolics that are easily arom-
atized into estrogen can cause a feminization of the breast tissue known
as gynecomastia. While largely dose related, a natural propensity for this
condition can cause it to occur even in moderate dosages. This condition
can often be avoided or arrested by the judicious use of anti-estrogenic
compounds. Once a serious cosmetic problem exists, minor surgery is required to correct it. Numerous professional bodybuilders have had this
surgery and others obviously need it (look closely at a very top place fin-
isher in the 1998 Mr. Olympia lineup).

Anabolic steroids and the liver

Anabolic steroids are processed by the liver. C-17 alkylated oral steroids
(steroids with an alkyl group added at the alpha position of the "C-17" or
number 17 carbon atom of the molecule to withstand total degradation
on their first pass through the liver) are unusually harsh on the liver. For
this reason, even moderate short-term administration of these C-17 oral
steroids can effect liver function test readings. Elevated liver counts indicating liver stress (toxicity) have been reported in recent studies of some-
what moderate oral anabolic steroid therapy (daily doses of 40 and 80 mg
of oxandrolone [Oxandrin, formerly Anavar]) as reported in the online
periodical *Medibolics,* edited by Michael Mooney (www.medibolics.com).
However, these elevated liver function readings will return to normal after cessation of a moderate, short-term steroid cycle. I could find not one
case to the contrary. Further, it is recognized that intense weight training
alone often causes changes in liver function tests, including SGOT, SGPT
and LDH (this is something that all physicians monitoring athletes using
anabolics should be familiar with).

---

*While normal guys will train more aggressively [on
steroids], they won't generally become violent.*

The more serious liver problems attributed to anabolic steroid use include hepatocellular carcinoma (liver cancer) and peliosis hepatitis
(blood-filled sacs within the liver). But the majority of cases reporting
liver problems have dealt with extremely sick and elderly patients treated
with C-17 alkylated oral steroids for years of continuous use, and many
of these patients had a particular type of anemia linked to liver tumors
even without anabolic steroid therapy. A computer search of the medical
literature looking for steroid-associated liver tumors could find only three
in athletes. Of the three athletes, one was using 700 mg of oxymetholone
a week for five straight years, and one had a tumor more indicative of
classic liver cancer than of steroid-associated tumors. Virtually all of the
reported liver problems seemed to occur with the 17 alpha-alkylated oral
steroids. There have been no cysts or liver tumors reported in athletes us-

ing the 17 beta-esterified injectable steroids. It has been noted that injectable steroids generally appear to have little effect on the liver at all.

Recent studies continue to suggest that reports of serious adverse effects of anabolic steroids upon the liver in healthy athletes may be highly overstated. In a study of athletes, of the 53 current or past steroid users who underwent laboratory testing, only one subject displayed an abnormal liver test (incidentally, on physical examination, not one user displayed evidence of any major abnormalities possibly attributable to steroids, such as high blood pressure, edema, acne or hair loss.) Another study tested one of the most powerful and reputedly dangerously toxic anabolic steroids for 30 weeks on HIV positive men and women. Oxymetholone, formerly known as Anadrol in the U.S. and a C-17 alkylated oral steroid, was administered in a dosage of over 1,000 mg per week (more than that used by many bodybuilders, and for a much longer duration of uninterrupted use). The results were significant gains in lean muscle mass—even without any weightlifting. Even more importantly—and surprisingly—there were no significant problems with liver function, water retention, or virilization side effects (it will be interesting to see whether further studies yield consistent findings at such high dosages).

While the dangers of anabolics to athletes' livers appear to have been highly exaggerated, it must be recognized that an apparently healthy athlete with a previously existing but undiscovered liver problem could do serious damage to himself by self-administering C-17 oral anabolic steroids. For this reason alone, it would be quite irresponsible for any athlete to use anabolic steroids without having a physician regularly conduct blood tests to monitor liver function.

Anabolic steroids and the heart

How cardiac risk might be increased by the use of steroids is a subject of speculation and some controversy. High blood pressure is perhaps "one of the most exaggerated claims" of steroid-related health risks [according to K.E. Friedl], and remains unconfirmed despite numerous studies. Regarding blood lipid levels, oral steroids in particular seem to cause a reduction in HDL (high-density lipoprotein cholesterol) levels in some steroid users. However, changes in the blood lipid levels now appear to begin to recover within about a month after discontinued use, and, in fact, most studies do not report an increase in total cholesterol.

In examining cardiovascular risks, often cited is a case report by R.A. McNutt, et al, 1988, concerning a 22-year-old steroid-using weightlifter who experienced a sudden heart attack. While often held out by anti-steroid authorities as the "smoking gun" connecting steroid use to heart attacks, a reading of the actual report reveals that the subject weighed 330 pounds and had a total serum cholesterol of a whopping 596 mg/dl! The fact that so few similar case studies exist may well indicate that the condition of this individual was hardly representative of the majority of athletes who use steroids. Nonetheless, all strength athletes, including steroid users, should regularly monitor serum cholesterol. Obviously, this poor fellow didn't get his cholesterol to 596 overnight, and it is not reported when he last visited a physician prior to his heart attack. To what extent our nation's criminalization approach to steroids, which discourages steroid-users from seeing doctors, contributed to this result is open to speculation.

While the question of whether short-term, reversible alterations of these cardiac risk factors are detrimental to long-term cardiac health is "unanswered" at this time, it has been suggested that some characteristics of steroid-users—intense exercising, low body fat, and avoidance of smoking—tend to put them in a low-risk group for heart disease.

Based on our present information, cardiac risks seem to be primarily related to high dosages in the absence of physician monitoring. Jose Antonio, PhD., a nationally recognized authority on drugs in sports who has written a monthly column for *Flex* magazine, cites a study examining serious cardiovascular side effects in four weightlifters using "massive amounts" of steroids. While there is little doubt that the health problems of these men were caused by their anabolic steroid abuse, these were clearly mega-dose abusers. "[H]igh dose equals high risk," notes Dr. Antonio, but "low-dose androgens (e.g., 200–600 mg per week for 10 weeks) pose little threat to health."

Anabolic steroids and the prostate

A legitimate concern is the potential adverse effect of excessive androgens on the prostate gland. While there is one case report of prostate cancer in a bodybuilder, no studies have shown an increased risk or incidence of prostatic cancer or hypertrophy with androgen use or indicated that androgens per se predispose to these conditions. Numerous male contraceptive studies using up to 200 mg/week for over a year show no evidence of prostate stimulation. Researchers at the University of Iowa recently examined the prostate effects of the administration for 15 weeks of up to 500 mg/week to healthy men in their twenties and thirties. No changes in prostate size or serum prostate specific antigen (PSA) levels were detected either during or up to 25 weeks after the last dose. Further, androgens are not the only or even the main causative factor in prostate cancer, as evinced by a case study in which a chronically testosterone deficient man developed prostate cancer. Warning: this does not necessarily mean that much higher dosages, especially of highly androgenic compounds, might not adversely effect the prostate, especially in older men. It is not known if athletes who have used steroids for prolonged periods will encounter more prostatic problems as they age.

Anabolic steroids and aggressive/psychiatric symptoms

Enormous media attention has been focused upon the reported adverse psychiatric effects (especially violent behavior) of steroid use. "Roid rage" is the descriptive term for steroid-induced "spontaneous, highly aggressive, out-of-control behavior where the police either were called or should have intervened," [according to Charles Yesalis and Virginia Cowart]. A few researchers have suggested that psychiatric symptoms including increased aggression are a common side effect of anabolic steroid use. For example, a flawed 1988 study suggested that psychiatric disorders occur with unusual frequency among athletes using anabolics. But the conclusions of these researchers have been regarded with skepticism by other experts. "If this phenomenon is real, it is relatively rare (probably less than 1 percent) among steroid users. Even among those affected, the impact of previous mental illness or abuse of other drugs is still unclear," [according to Charles Yesalis and Virginia Cowart]. "Some long-time steroid users have never suffered any emotional instability, or anything more than transient physical effects" and many steroid users describe non-violent feelings of euphoria, well-being and enhanced self-confidence as common effects, [according to J.E. Wright and Virginia Cowart]. In one study [conducted by M.S. Bahrke et al.] to determine the psychiatric effects of steroid use on athletes, no significant differences could be found between users and non-users. "The facts that steroids have been used by tens of thousands if not hundreds of thousands of athletes over two decades and that behavioral effects are only recently being discovered (in small numbers) tend to support [that feelings of aggression may not be observed in the majority of steroid users]. Our findings are compatible with and complementary to those in anecdotal reports and data from individual psychiatrists." The researchers do not rule out, however, the possibility that in a small minority of predisposed individuals, "steroid use may be sufficient to push them over the edge and contribute to irrational or violent behavior." Many experienced steroid users have found that steroids enhance certain preexisting personality problems. Angry and combative users will become angrier and more combative; however, while normal guys will train more aggressively, they won't generally become violent.

Despite over forty years of use by athletes, . . . we have yet to hear reports of an epidemic of steroid-related deaths.

Not surprisingly, when psychiatric problems do occur in study subjects, there seems to be a direct correlation between dosage and prevalence of syndromes. For example, no significant psychiatric effects have been noted where reported mean weekly dosage was 318 mg (heaviest user was 620 mg/wk). But where reported dosage exceeded 1,000 mg/wk, 11 out of 25 subjects (44%) exhibited mood disorders. While, based on this and other studies, there is a dose-related correlation between steroid use and psychiatric effects, it must be noted that not all steroid users exhibit such symptoms; in fact, nearly 90% of light and moderate dosage users in this particular study exhibited no mood disorder symptoms at all.

The psychiatric effect that massive amounts of anabolics might have upon predisposed individuals has created a new defense in criminal cases. Just as voluntary alcohol intoxication can be used to negate the specific intent required for certain crimes, so has voluntary ingestion of anabolic steroids been offered in the defense of various violent crimes in an effort to prove that the accused was unable to distinguish right from wrong or to understand the consequences of his acts. A sampling of these cases reveals, generally, that such defenses were unsuccessfully raised. This may be due in part to the fact that in many cases the dosages administered were either not specified or were too low to be persuasive. A bigger factor may be the general reluctance of juries to acquit in murder cases based on insanity defenses, especially where the insanity was caused by a voluntarily consumed substance.

Anabolic steroids and psychological dependence

There is some evidence that anabolic steroid use can lead to psychological dependence in certain individuals. Whether the dependence is due to chemical effects upon the brain or simply because of the positive reinforcement occasioned by a more muscular physique is not known. Whatever the cause, this may be the most dangerous aspect of steroid use for those it affects. The cessation of steroid use, especially after a prolonged cycle, often leaves the user in a state of low endogenous testosterone levels. For individuals with an inadequate sense of self, the loss of some portion of the steroid gains can be psychologically devastating to the ego. These individuals can be unable to resist immediately resuming steroid use. Further, as the goal of hardcore bodybuilders is not optimal muscle size, but maximal muscle size, dosages can become excessive. While many athletes successfully use steroids intermittently and with moderation, it is a sobering thought that there are certain individuals who start out on low risk, short-term cycles and ultimately end up using massive dosages for years of uninterrupted use. It might be theorized that the problem of dependence on steroids by certain bodybuilders has less to do with the nature of the substance than with the psychological profile of the users.

Other adverse effects of anabolic steroids

• *Connective tissue injuries.* The medical literature regarding the suggestion of increased athletic injuries caused by anabolic steroid use is scant. It is not unreasonable to expect muscle and tendon tears in hardcore strength athletes, regardless of steroid use. However, the exceptional frequency and severity (often requiring surgical reattachment) of such injuries in professional level bodybuilders do raise suspicions as to the possibility that steroids, diuretics, or other drugs may be implicated. Former Mr. Olympia Dorian Yates has suffered training-related injuries to the chest, leg and biceps, and retired after a major triceps injury. Pro bodybuilder Alq Gurley reportedly completely tore the quadriceps muscles in both legs when he fell while simply walking! Whether these injuries are steroid-related is as yet unknown, although some animal studies have suggested that steroids may cause tendon degeneration and increased risk of tendon rupture. It may not be unreasonable to assume that, like many adverse steroid effects, connective tissue injuries are mostly associated with high-dose, prolonged usage.

• *AIDS.* Many articles include this as a possible consequence. Quite frankly, anyone who would even consider sharing needles with his gym buddies in this day and age is so irresponsible and judgment-impaired that the substance of this entire article is lost on him.

• *Premature Closure of Growth Plates.* Chronic steroid usage prior to puberty or in early adolescence can cause premature closure of the growth plates of the long bones, preventing the young user from attaining full natural height. For this reason as well as others previously discussed, teenagers should not use steroids for muscle building.

The dangers of counterfeit steroids

One of the primary effects of our government's crackdown on legitimate anabolic steroids has been the expansion of a huge black market of counterfeit products. While estimates vary widely, many authorities assert that the majority of anabolics available on the black market are fakes. These counterfeits are manufactured under unsupervised and potentially unsanitary conditions, and may contain no real androgens at all. They may also be contaminated with bacteria or other dangerous substances. Noted steroid expert Dr. Robert Price: "My colleagues at Mount Sinai Hospital in New York tell me they are treating many more athletes for side effects of counterfeit and bogus steroids than they did when reliable pharmacy-purchased steroids were available."

If the health dangers of real anabolic steroids have been overstated, the dangers of counterfeit anabolics may be understated. The problem is particularly serious because of how difficult it is to distinguish a real product from a counterfeit knock-off. . . .

It can be concluded that "[a]s used by most athletes, the side effects of anabolic steroid use appear to be minimal," [according to M.G. DiPasquale]. Despite over forty years of use by athletes, many of whom are now well into middle-age, we have yet to hear reports of an epidemic of steroid-related deaths. A review of the medical literature does not support the depiction of a serious health crisis related to anabolic steroids. Of course, it would be untrue to say that anabolic steroids, especially black market products, are safe for unsupervised, unmonitored self-administration. On the other hand, it would be equally untrue to say that anabolics are "deadly drugs" deserving of the imposition of harsh criminal penalties for personal use by adults. Accordingly, there is a serious question as to whether Congress may have grossly overreacted in addressing the non-medical use of anabolic steroids by athletes.

12

One Strike, You're Out

Mark Starr

Mark Starr is a sports columnist for Newsweek *magazine.*

Olympic officials have begun to take the widespread abuse of performance-enhancing drugs by Olympic athletes seriously. The crackdown comes in response to fears that fans and sponsors will no longer support the Olympics if drug scandals become a regular feature of the Games. Newly established anti-doping agencies have increased the investment in drug tests designed to keep pace with drug cheats, who continually use new drugs and masking agents to beat the tests. A successful program of random drug testing was also introduced prior to the 2002 Winter Olympics in Salt Lake City, leaving drug-using athletes with less opportunity to render their drug intake undetectable before competitions.

Ludmila Engquist dreamed of making Olympic history by becoming the first woman ever to win gold medals at both the summer and winter games. Engquist, a Russian-born Swede, had won the 100-meter hurdles in Atlanta in 1996. Now she was taking aim at gold again, this time around in the inaugural women's bobsled competition at the Salt Lake City Olympics next February.

But this week Engquist made history a bit prematurely—and not in glory on the Olympic–medal podium, but rather in sad, even tragic, fashion. She became the first Olympic athlete, man or woman, who has ever been caught using illegal drugs in two different sports.

Back in 1993, Engquist tested positive for steroids at a track meet and was banned from competition for four years. But a Russian court cleared her when her husband claimed he had spiked her protein powder as revenge after she filed for divorce. After two years, her suspension was lifted by the international track federation, enabling her to triumph in Atlanta. Her defense was typical of virtually every Olympic athlete ever caught with drugs in their system: first denials; then challenges of the testing procedures; finally, insistence that the illegal substance must have been in their diet supplement or that their Coca-Cola was spiked. Or perhaps a Neptunian drifted down from outer space one night and injected them while they slept. No athlete ever simply fessed up and said, "OK. You caught me. I did it. I'm guilty. I'm sorry."

Which means that Engquist made another sort of history, too. Because this time she, so to speak, came clean. Caught in a random test before a practice run in Norway, Engquist later faxed a letter to the Swedish news agency TT, saying, "I took drugs secretly . . . I did something terrible and I feel terribly bad." At least as remarkable was the fact that Engquist confessed to using steroids before the test had actually been analyzed, which means she must have been caught, at least metaphorically, with the needle practically in her arm. Engquist had been widely admired as something of a heroic figure in track when she took a bronze medal in the 1999 world championships just a few months after undergoing a mastectomy and chemotherapy for breast cancer. In the fax, she said she was so distraught at being caught cheating that she had attempted suicide.

Olympic officials realize that . . . the scourge of illegal, performance-enhancing drugs remains the greatest threat of all.

In the wake of the Sept. 11 terrorist attacks, no subject concerning the impending Salt Lake Olympics will be discussed more than security. The International Olympic Committee as well as U.S. and Salt Lake Olympic officials will all repeat again and again, quite truthfully, that the safety of the athletes and spectators is paramount in their minds. But Olympic officials realize that, in the long run, the scourge of illegal, performance-enhancing drugs remains the greatest threat of all. After a succession of scandals—from East Germany to China, from sprinter Ben Johnson to Irish swimmer Michelle Smith to American shot-putter C.J. Hunter—most Olympic insiders believe that drug abuse remains rampant in Olympic competition. If the fans ever truly catch on to the dimensions of the problem, they will turn off, sponsors will flee and the world's biggest athletic empire will crumble.

To the extent that fans are aware of the drug problem, they tend to associate it with the summer Olympics, most notably with swimming and track and field. But it is epidemic at the Winter Olympics, as well, especially in sports that Americans regard as minor such as bobsled, speedskating and Nordic skiing. Earlier this year a misplaced medical bag led to a scandal that rocked Finland, where its Nordic skiing stars were viewed as every bit as pristine as the surface they traversed. The bag, belonging to the Finnish Ski Association, contained needles, syringes and drugs used to manipulate blood-cell counts. Six Finnish skiing stars were eventually banned from competition for two years after testing positive for an illegal substance often used to mask the human growth hormone EPO. Among them was Harri Kirvesniemi, a Finnish legend who has competed in six Olympics and won 11 medals.

For years now, it has taken just such a freak occurrence to expose widespread cheating. With drug testing largely restricted to competition medallists, "the only athlete you could catch was the dumb one," says Terry Madden, the CEO of the U.S. Anti-Doping Agency (USADA), the new independent agency that will handle American compliance. While this country leads the world in finger-pointing, it has not pursued its own athletes with any particular vigor. And when American athletes have been caught, authorities here have usually taken the same charitable view of their denials and convoluted explanations as the Russian court did with Engquist, indeed as virtually every country does with its own.

But with an endless succession of scandals, the recognition of the potential threat to the Olympic movement and some increased political pressure, the international community is finally paying more than lip service to the matter. A Toronto-based worldwide antidoping agency, similar to the new American one, has been established. With them has finally come some significant financial investment in new drug tests that could challenge the conventional wisdom that the cheaters, with their resources, will always be at least one step ahead in developing new drugs and masking agents. "The belief has always been that we can never change this," says Gen. Barry McCaffrey, who as U.S. drug czar was highly critical of the enforcement efforts in athletics. "But it looks like in the coming 10 years—if the international cooperation continues on the science and the political will is maintained to enforce—we could see a major change."

Along with the science, the key change is the implementation of a massive program of random testing. Sophisticated coaches and athletes can manage a drug regimen that is invisible by the time of competitions. But if enforcement's new mantra becomes "any time, anywhere," the risk-reward equation is seriously altered. Approximately 75 percent of the athletes coming to compete in Salt Lake will have been tested in the past year, but only about a third of those tests will have been random. By Athens, enforcement officials are hopeful that 100 percent of all competitors will have undergone tests with at least half of those random. "For a long time now the clean athletes have been feeling at both a physiological and psychological disadvantage," says the USADA's Madden. "We're turning that around and giving back the clean athlete the advantage."

It is also essential that the various international and national governing bodies stick to a no-tolerance policy. "If it's in your system, then you're guilty," says Madden. The athlete must be responsible for what's in their body, thus relieving enforcers of the impossible task of sorting out the truths, half-truths and lies. Some athletes may be innocently tainted, but that's the only way to target the far greater number of cheats. That's why, as unfair as it may have seemed at the time, it was right to strip 16-year-old Romanian gymnast Andrea Raducan of her gold medal in Sydney—even if, as she insisted, the illegal stimulant was taken unwittingly in an over-the-counter cold medication and may not even have been beneficial to her performance.

Some experts remain skeptical of both the commitment of the international athletic community and its ability to catch, as well as catch up to, the cheaters. But this week, as Engquist was confessing her guilt, the suspension of a world-ranked American swimmer, Michael Picotte, was also announced. His suspension came after he refused to take an out-of-competition test. The game has changed for Olympic hopefuls. And finally, thankfully, it's one strike, and you're out.

13

Performance-Enhancing Drug Testing Is Ineffective

Anonymous

The author was intimately involved in drug testing for a variety of sports.

The International Olympic Committee and other sports organizations use ineffective performance-enhancing drug testing techniques and remain insincere about catching drug-using athletes. Claims that drug use is declining as a result of tougher testing, as evidenced by the low number of positive drug test results, are false, since there are many methods that athletes can employ to beat drug tests. In addition, athletes with access to money and support personnel stand a better chance of passing the tests than athletes who lack such resources, making the drug testing system unfair.

If I told you I was committed to an effort and was going to spend one million dollars of my money on a project, wouldn't that seem like a sincere effort? Now let's say you find out from a reliable source that the one million dollars represents mere pennies to me because I have tons of money. Then you find out that the project I was supposedly committed to is last on my funding list as far as financial commitment. Does it still seem like a high priority? This is the case with drug testing. In general, the International Olympic Committee (IOC) and other organizations talk a good game, but in reality, they are not sincere in their drug testing efforts. The historical evidence shows a repeating sequence of events since the implementation of drug testing: athletes take drugs, organizations develop tests, athletes beat tests, organizations come out with new tests, athletes beat tests, and so on. You get the point. Each time a new test is developed, drug testing officials release statements to the media indicating how sensitive the new techniques are. The tests get implemented and a very small percentage of athletes test positive for some type of banned substance. The drug testing officials then claim that based on their latest information, drug use is declining. This is comical, given all the data that indicates junior high school, high school, recreational, amateur and professional athletes are using steroids and other drugs. Yet somehow the IOC and other organizations want us to believe that they are cleaning things up based on the low number of positive drug test results. Given all the data that indicates drug use is prevalent, I feel that what the low numbers of positive drug tests actually indicate is how inadequate drug testing methods are.

Basic overview of drug testing

Prohibited and restricted drugs fall into three main categories: (1) short- or immediate-acting stimulants and beta-blockers, (2) anabolic agents, and (3) masking agents. Stimulants and beta-blockers tend to affect performance only if taken just before the event. Drug testing for this category of drugs is believed to be very effective. Based on drug testing data, stimulant use has been essentially abolished from high-level sports because they are detected so easily. Anabolic agents usually require weeks to obtain the desired effect and are sometimes referred to as training drugs. The training drugs are inherently more difficult to detect and can be discontinued in time to pass an announced or anticipated test. Masking agents are drugs that affect the detectability of other drugs. Examples of masking agents are diuretics, probenecid, and epitestosterone. These drugs are only useful at the time of the test and, except for epitestosterone, are relatively easy to detect. . . .

What the low numbers of positive drug tests actually indicate is how inadequate drug testing methods are.

On an annual basis, over 100,000 drug tests are conducted worldwide at a cost of $30 million. The drug tests are designed to detect and deter abuse of performance-enhancing drugs by competitors. The testing procedures for drug abuse in sport are strict and at times deemed unfair. They are deemed unfair because athletes are responsible for knowing what is banned despite the fact that additions are made almost daily to the list of banned substances. This has prompted researchers to recommend to athletes that the best possible solution is to avoid all drugs unless listed on the allowed substance list. The IOC has decided that drug tests will require confirmation, whenever possible, by gas chromatography and mass spectrometry, which define several chemical features of an abused drug, in effect producing a drug fingerprint. In addition, prior to the 1996 Olympic Games in Atlanta, the IOC required competitors to agree to a contract that prohibited them from taking any action beyond arbitration if they failed a drug test.

When athletes know when a drug test will occur, they can prepare for it and thereby neutralize the effects of drug testing on the use of performance-enhancing drugs and/or masking agents. Year-round short-notice and no-notice testing are the most effective means to curtail the use of training drugs because they make athletes always at risk to be tested. Sports have recently begun to invest in this type of testing despite the high cost and difficulty in administration. Some countries claim to have achieved no-notice testing. The International Association of Athletics Federations (IAAF) and international federations for swimming and weightlifting conduct year-round, short-notice testing. In the United States, the National Collegiate Athletic Association (NCAA) and the National Football League (NFL) have short-notice (1–2 days) programs, and the United States Olympic Committee (USOC) has approved the implementation of a no-notice program.

Obtaining a urine sample

The drug testing procedure begins with taking a urine sample. While this sounds simple, it initiates a formal and highly regulated procedure to ensure that the urine sample that arrives at the laboratory actually comes from the athlete in question, with no opportunity to tamper with the sample. Why is urine used and not blood or other tissues? There are several reasons. Blood draws would require medical or paramedical staff and hence incur additional costs.[1] Other tissues may not be valid for analysis under all conditions. Once selected for drug testing, the athlete is notified by an official and asked to sign a form acknowledging this notification. The athlete may or may not be accompanied by an official and must attend the testing station within the designated period. The testing station is supposed to be a private, comfortable place where plenty of drinks are available. Many times it is set up inside a specially designed mobile testing unit. Independent sampling officers, whom are trained and appointed by the respective governing body, carry out the collection of urine samples. Each officer carries a time-limited identity card and a letter of authority for the event to which they are allocated.

The whole idea behind drug testing is to have a level playing field. Yet, in reality, this system is inherently unfair.

Before giving a urine sample, the athlete is told to select two numbered bottles. After providing the sample (about 100 ml), the athlete must voluntarily complete a form. The athlete declares any drug treatment taken in the previous seven days and must check and sign that the sample has been taken and placed in the bottles correctly. The urine sample is then sent for analysis to a laboratory currently accredited by the IOC. In the event of a positive test result, the laboratory will notify the governing body of the sport, who will then notify the athlete. The rules of the governing body of the particular sport determine what happens next. The rules vary across governing bodies, sports, and countries. An athlete is usually suspended while a positive result is investigated, but has the right to have a second analysis of the urine sample. This analysis may be observed directly by the athlete or by the athlete's representative. There follows a hearing, at which time the athlete's case is presented. An appeal can be made, and there have been successful appeals both in the United States and other countries. . . .

---

1. Blood testing was introduced at the 2000 Sydney Olympic Games for the banned drug erythropoietin (EPO).

At the elite level, athletes are subject to year-round random testing. At any time, an independent sampling officer may call unannounced and request a urine sample. While this comes across straightforward on paper, in practice there are many difficulties. Frequently, athletes travel the world and finding the athlete can be difficult. After the independent sampling officer asks around to find the athlete in question, it is unlikely that the testing remains a surprise. . . .

Beating drug tests

The dosages of anabolic-androgenic steroids (AAS) that athletes take greatly exceed the normal therapeutic amounts and typically several different types of AAS are taken together (stacked) or used at different times (cycled). Most athletes use AAS as training aids for recovery and discontinue use before an event so that they can later pass the competition drug test. During a typical steroid cycle, it is common for athletes to use other drugs such as diuretics to reduce fluid retention, thyroxine to promote weight loss, and tamoxifen to prevent gynecomastia. In the US and other countries, these agents are freely available in gyms and fitness clubs, regardless of their legal status.

Athletes with access to the right resources can beat the drug tests. Other athletes can not. The whole idea behind drug testing is to have a level playing field. Yet, in reality, this system is inherently unfair. If one athlete has the money and appropriate support personnel around them, they could certainly challenge a test. If another athlete has little money and knowledge, they will be at a serious disadvantage.

About 2–3 years before working as a drug test official, I was at a party being thrown by some collegiate athletes. People were lighting up joints everywhere and drinking alcohol like crazy. I knew my one buddy was going to get drug tested, because he was a big guy (almost 300 pounds) and he was always tested. Even though he wasn't smoking anything (at least at that party) he wasn't worried. He said he never tested positive for marijuana even though he got stoned plenty of times the night before a drug test. He figured that because he was so big he just got rid of any residues really fast. While that didn't make that much sense to me, the fact was that he still had negative lab results. Based on the formal proceedings this didn't seem possible. This became clear to me years later.

A loophole in college drug tests

If you ever saw the movie "The Program," then you were treated to the various non-chemical means by which athletes have tried to beat the drug tests. I have seen or heard of athletes getting caught trying to use someone else's urine by planting hidden vials in the bathroom, keeping a plastic bag and a catheter down their pants, etc. I have never seen or heard of collegiate athletes infusing someone else's urine into their own bladder in order to beat the drug test. I have heard of this at the professional and elite levels of competition, though. To get around all the mechanical methods that athletes used to beat AAS tests, several key checks were done on every urine sample, as it was produced. By 1995, the procedure had evolved to the following: an athlete goes into his locker room and sees a notice on his locker to show up for drug testing. The notices were supposed to be put out right before practice, so the athlete knows not to use the bathroom. After practice the athlete shows up to the drug test site, which was usually in or near the locker room. From that point on the athlete has a monitor assigned to him. The athlete selects his own container to urinate in. ID labels are placed on the cup and on other documents. The athlete and monitor go to the bathroom where the athlete urinates in front of the monitor. The monitor must witness the flow of urine into the specimen container. After the appropriate volume is collected and capped, the athlete and monitor return to the drug-testing site where documentation is completed and signed by the athlete. At this time, the pH, temperature, and specific gravity of the urine are measured using indicator strips on the sample container. (This would serve to eliminate the use of vials of urine and prevent tampering with the actual urine sample.) If all of the three measurements are within the appropriate range, then the athlete can sign off and leave. If even one is off, then another sample must be collected.

It was totally possible that . . . small or thin looking athletes could use steroids and never get caught, even though he was drug tested.

That was the routine stuff that the athlete saw. Now let's talk about what really happens with the urine results. NCAA athletes are told that they will be tested for cocaine, marijuana, AAS, and amphetamines. They are led to believe that each sample will be tested for each and every drug. Remember my big buddy who never tested positive for marijuana? The reason is simple: they never tested his urine for marijuana. The rule of thumb that I learned years later was as follows: Since drug testing costs so much, the big guys like linemen, fullbacks, and shot putters would be tested for steroids, while smaller guys would be tested for other drugs, like marijuana. So to spell it out, it was totally possible that a wide receiver, light-weight wrestler, or some other small or thin looking athletes could use steroids and never get caught, even though he was drug tested. On the other hand, a lineman could get stoned all the time and theoretically not test positive for marijuana or cocaine because they always tested his urine for steroids.

Weightlifting and drug use

If you've followed weightlifting for years then you know how dominant the Bulgarian weightlifting team once was. How were they able to compete at the international level so successfully? I'll say it for you: DRUGS. Never mind all of the bullshit with training and restorative means. Today they still have access to the same type of training and recovery methods, yet they are not nearly as dominant as they once were. The reason that the Bulgarians were able to train six times per day at very high intensities and make consistent progress is that they had figured out how to hide their drug use. While they used a variety of tricks, here are some of the methods we have been able to verify. The Bulgarian weightlifting team would fast about 2–3 days before a competition. Fasting lowers the amplitude and pulsatility of luteinizing hormone. This, in turn, would lower endogenous production of testosterone (T). In addition, fasting also causes an increase in the excretion of steroids. As a result, their urine samples would show lower levels of T and other steroids because by the time they were tested, they virtually excreted most of the evidence away. Now this trick was not the only one the Bulgarians were known for. Their real ace in the hole was the use of diuretics. They would use the diuretics to urinate out lots of fluid. By ingesting an abundance of water, the diuretics would just accelerate the clearance of steroids or other banned substances from the blood. This offered two advantages: the first was that now the athlete would avoid detection for a banned substance and the second was that the athlete could lose weight and compete at a lighter weight class. But the diuretics proved to be their downfall, as this is how they got caught. At one Olympics, the whole team was forced to withdraw from competition because every member of the lighter weight classes had tested positive for diuretics. To avoid further embarrassment, the rest of the team was withdrawn. So next time someone tells you about what the Bulgarians do for training, slap them in the face and wake them up. Then remind them that Bulgaria is not the dominant power it once was in weightlifting. The only thing that changed was that the drug testing got better.

Athletes can, and always will, maintain a few paces ahead of drug-testing efforts.

So how about the boys from the US? Are they clean? Clean is such an ambiguous term, so let's be more precise: Are they taking anabolic-androgenic steroids? I have never seen or heard about first-hand any athlete on the Olympic team using AAS (we all know about the 1976 athletes and subsequent athletes testing positive). However, I have heard of AAS, growth hormone, and other agents, being used by lower caliber athletes. I also know of athletes that took prohormones and tested negative. The tests, as far as I could tell, were complete and nothing like the "insurance policy or sink-test" type tests Dr. Voy has written about in his book [*Drugs, Sport, and Politics*] (where athletes' urine samples are dumped down a drain and then the results are reported as negative). These athletes did not use any type of strategies to avoid detection. There can be several reasons for the negative results. Perhaps the athletes ingested pills that did not contain sufficient quantities of DHEA or androstenedione (A). Perhaps the amounts of DHEA or A in the pills were not enough to result in a positive test. Lastly, maybe the conversion of androgens to estrogens is so rapid that the current tests can not detect the androgens (elevated urinary estrogen levels would not matter since these were not tested for). Typically athletes would take 100–200 mg of A before a workout. The rationalization was that the sudden elevation of T from the conversion of A would result in more aggressiveness and a better workout. While we may ponder whether or not these tactics work, consider what one athlete did with access to more sophisticated means. He simply designed his own "study" using himself as the sole subject. On different days he would take increasing dosages of DHEA, A or some combination. So one day he might take 100 mg of A, another day he might take 100 mg of DHEA and 100 mg of A, then another day he would take 200 mg of A, etc. He would have his blood hormone levels measured and his urine analyzed. He found that at around 800–1000 mg of A by itself, he could get enough of an increase in T to increase his training performance. If he was ever drug tested, the conversion of A to estrone (and T to estradiol) would also serve to lower his A and T levels, thus offering a "negative" urine sample. This may have worked for him, but other athletes should not be gullible and follow the same strategy. Unless they undergo the same type of self-study, they have no way of knowing if the androgen elevations and conversions will be the same for them. In short, you can not rely on another athlete's hormonal and urinary data and adopt it as your own.

Even before many tests are implemented, athletes are aware of the means to beat the test.

The less sophisticated athletes simply make use of the loop hole in USA Weightlifting's drug testing policy. An athlete has to be enrolled in their no-notice drug-testing program for at least six months prior to the local, regional, or national competition that would qualify the athlete for international competition. So you could take AAS for three years, get stronger and lift more, then enroll in the program after you come off, test negative, post a qualifying total, and then go on to international competition (providing of course you earn that right by lifting some big weights). This is not a slight against USA Weightlifting in any way, obviously there is no way you can know who to test before they tell you they wish to be considered for international competition. It merely points out that athletes can, and always will, maintain a few paces ahead of drug-testing efforts.

General methods used to avoid detection

The next series of tactics are not limited to any particular sport. They will be presented in terms of the rationale behind their use and what was done to prevent or curb their use. Initially when athletes were first exposed to drug testing, they were caught off guard. Analytical chemistry was not something most athletes specialized in. After consulting with more qualified personnel, coaches and athletes realized that simply going off AAS so that sufficient time would pass, thus clearing the AAS from their system, would result in a negative drug test. This was done by simply submitting urine samples to a lab with the appropriate analytical equipment. Each day the athlete would find out the results of the previous day's drug test. At some point he/she would know exactly how many days it would take to pass a drug test. Then going into a meet, the athlete would feel calm that they already knew the results and would test negative. This worked well until the introduction of different methods for AAS detection.

The uncertainty of not knowing which type of equipment would be used or the methods that would be followed created a demand by athletes for some other methods to avoid detection. As mentioned previously, diuretic use was one type of strategy. Diuretics have been abused in sports with weight classes and are used to shed weight quickly. (In the old days of powerlifting, it was common to see athletes using diuretics to make weight and then rehydrate using an intravenous drip.) Diuretics are also used to increase urine volume and dilution, thus making small quantities of banned substances more difficult to detect. Although drug testing started in 1976, it was not until 1988 that testing for diuretics began. So now with diuretics on the banned list, other alternatives had to be found. Physical methods such as catheterization and urine substitution continued to be practiced.

Perhaps the final war between athletes avoiding detection and drug testers will be in the legal system.

Alternatively, renal blocking agents were sought out. The premise is simple enough: If you can't urinate the conjugates and other metabolites of AAS out of your system, then you can't get caught. Probenecid was the most common offender in this category of agents. It retards the excretion of a variety of drugs, including AAS. Athletes taking masking agents could continue taking AAS closer to competition before discontinuing their use and still pass the drug tests. Once it was realized that athletes were using probenecid and related agents, these drugs were added to the banned substance list.

The use of testosterone is also another method for avoiding detection. At this time, the current methods do not distinguish between exogenous and endogenous testosterone. To control for this, drug testing includes standards for the detection of testosterone abuse, with a 6:1 ratio of testosterone (T) to its free analogue, epitestosterone (E). The ratio of T to E in the urine is normally less than two. Athletes responded to this test by simply taking epitestosterone in order to maintain the 6:1 ratio. So then of course, epitestosterone was added to the banned substance list.

Future trends

Research has been done on a variety of fronts to prevent and eliminate the use of banned substances. Unfortunately, even before many tests are implemented, athletes are aware of the means to beat the test. One such example is that the use of longitudinal data, in order to get an accurate hormonal profile of the athlete, has been investigated. If the urinary T:E ratio for an athlete is consistently in a given range and then increases beyond normal limits, may be an indication of substance use. While such testing has yet to be implemented, athletes are already using sublingual cyclodextrin-testosterone preparations. Such preparations allow the T:E ratio to return to normal within a few hours.

Another technique under investigation measures the ratio of the carbon isotopes C 12 and C 13 in testosterone and in two of the hormone's precursors contained in a urine sample. Research in this area suggests that the use of banned substances should be suspected when the ratios don't match. Endogenously produced T differs in the carbon isotope ratios from exogenously administered T, which is normally synthesized from plant sources. Again, athletes are a step ahead by using bovine/porcine/equine testosterone preparations, which are believed to contain carbon isotope ratios very similar to that of endogenous T.

It is believed that peptide hormones will be the most widely used banned substance in the 2000 Olympic games. None of these hormones can be detected with the existing International Olympic Committee methods. So before the games, GH2000, an international project hoping to develop a legally sound methodology to detect and validate use and abuse of exogenously administered growth hormone and related substances, was developed. Presently the detection methods are still undergoing validation and have not been implemented. Athletes have already been using GH nasal preparations, which once inhaled, have a very short half-life in the blood.

Perhaps the final war between athletes avoiding detection and drug testers will be in the legal system. Immunoassays for some drugs have been automated in order to keep the cost low for screening purposes. However, a positive result by immunoassay is by itself insufficient, so confirmation by a more accurate method is required. Gas chromatography combined with mass spectrometry is regarded as the reference method because the end result is a "fingerprint" for the drug or metabolite. The results are usually accepted as a high degree of evidence of the presence of a compound. The weak link lies in the fact that the equipment is very expensive and the interpretation of the data requires a great degree of skill. When labs subcontract out labor for drug testing, it may be possible to get a poorly skilled individual interpreting the data. While researches may agree that an athlete was using a banned substance, legally an attorney could raise sufficient suspicion as to the validity of the results, ultimately allowing the athlete to "beat" the test.

14

Performance-Enhancing Dietary Supplements Are Dangerous

Gwen Knapp

Gwen Knapp is a sports journalist for the San Francisco Chronicle.

Athletes are using dietary supplements purchased from health-food stores to boost their athletic performance. Many of these products are advertised as having the same effects on muscle development as prescription-only performance-enhancing drugs, and studies have shown that some supplements convert to illicit steroids once ingested. Supplement use has been linked to the deaths of several athletes, who exceeded the recommended dosages or mixed their intake of supplements with other medications. Because the supplement industry is virtually unregulated due to a 1994 law passed by Congress, consumers should use caution when purchasing performance-enhancing dietary supplements.

O pen up the liquor cabinets. Turn over the car keys. And—what the heck?—hand out cigarettes for Halloween.

No age limits on supplement sales

If an 11-year-old tennis player can walk into an alleged health-food store and legally purchase something called Ripped Fuel, which often comes in canisters showing a man's torso covered with bulging ribbons of muscle, then why not let her light up?

If a youth-baseball coach can distribute androstenedione, famed as [Major League Baseball player] Mark McGwire's hinky alternative to Wheaties, without a word of dissent from the police, why not let the kids unwind with a cold six-pack after the game?

In the unchecked market for nutritional supplements, there are virtually no limits. Athletes have been drawn to this stuff as if it were Michael Jordan's latest shoe model. Ultimate Orange, Ripped Fuel, Xenadrine—they're as easy to buy as toothpaste.

A few years ago, a certain chain of vitamin stores refused to stock androstenedione [andro] because of its uncertain safety record. The stuff was banned at the Olympics, and the stores decided that was a sufficiently negative endorsement.

Then it was reported that McGwire took andro during his record-breaking, home-run binge in 1998, and it became the must-have ingredient of the late-'90s. The stores then started dealing.

Athletes have been drawn to [dietary supplements] as if it were Michael Jordan's latest shoe model.

Summer 2001's headlines belong to ephedra, a stimulant and weight-loss aid found in some popular supplements. Rashidi Wheeler, the Northwestern safety who died in August 2001 after preseason drills, had ephedra in his system, according to a coroner's report. Two other football players who died during the summer of 2001—Davaughn Darling of Florida State and Curtis Jones, a defensive lineman in an indoor football league—reportedly had used supplements containing ephedra.

Officially, an asthma attack killed Wheeler. Several doctors have pointed out that taking ephedra with asthma medication, or simply with a case of asthma, made for a dangerous combination. But the medical examiner said that ephedra was not specifically the cause of death; so, its hands are clean. Don't be shocked now if the coroner's report turns up in promotional material for Wheeler's supplement of choice.

Every month or so, my e-mail contains ads for "Legal bodybuilding anabolics!"—"Hard to obtain pharmaceuticals." The ad, in its entirety, promises substances that duplicate steroidal effects legally, because the knockoffs don't require a prescription.

Charles Yesalis, a professor of health and human development at Penn State, has researched performance-enhancing drugs for 23 years, and he has become a crusader against steroids. He doesn't have any simple solutions for the mania around supplements.

Ephedra turns up in diet pills, in decongestants sold over the counter. Most Americans have taken it, and if they want to ramp up the dosage and risk their health, Yesalis is uncomfortable telling them to stop.

"If somebody runs a magazine ad promising a substance that can make me look like Mark McGwire and make you look like Faith Hill, and we fall for it, that's our fault," Yesalis said. "It's not the government's job to stop adults from making morons of themselves."

Supplements skirt regulation

The problem with the supplements is that they are virtually unregulated. In 1994, Congress passed a law that says the Food and Drug Administration has to keep its hands off dietary supplements unless a brand has already caused serious harm. In other words, we are all guinea pigs.

For sports teams, this is a dilemma. If you're a college trainer, you can refuse to deal with the supplements, but then you abdicate control over what athletes are taking and how much. Some trainers think it's wiser to hand out creatine [an amino acid sold as a supplement] rather than let athletes find the stuff on their own.

In the past two years, more and more international athletes have tested positive for nandrolone and argued that they had no idea they were taking a banned drug. At least four studies of ostensibly legal supplements have shown that some of them contain a substance that converts to nandrolone, an illicit steroid, once it is digested.

Yet the same legislators who won't allow marijuana use for cancer patients cover their eyes and ears on this subject. Campaign contributions from the industry might have dulled their appetite for a fight.

Yesalis tells parents to lobby for the firing of any coach who advocates supplement use for minors. But he knows that families can't protect youngsters from themselves, from the urge to take pills they shouldn't, to take 10 when only one is recommended.

Wheeler was 22 when he died, old enough to vote, drink and smoke. But if he had been 20, too young for alcohol, he still could have legally downed a supplement that doesn't carry the same nutritional statistics found on a can of Coke.

Some supplement manufacturers do include warnings on their packages, insisting that a product is designed only for people of certain age, and often exclusively for men. But right now, the best hope for placing limits on this industry lies with the one group that can make money off tragedies.

Product-liability lawyers will have to play sheriff. And if that means attorneys have to chase an athlete's ambulance, let's just hope they're running as fast as someone on Ripped Fuel.

15

Performance-Enhancing Dietary Supplements Are Safe

Council for Responsible Nutrition

The Council for Responsible Nutrition is a trade association represent-ing the dietary supplement industry.

Performance-enhancing dietary supplements like creatine and ephedra are safe when used by healthy people within the recom-mended dosage limits. Media assertions that supplements are un-regulated as a result of the 1994 Dietary Supplement Health and Education Act are false—the Food and Drug Administration (FDA) has the authority to regulate supplements in the same way that it regulates any other food product. The FDA should exercise its reg-ulatory authority constructively to increase consumer confidence in dietary supplements.

It is human nature to seek an "edge" to support and improve perfor-mance, and sports supplements are one tool millions of people have found helpful. As with all efforts to improve health and increase perfor-mance, common sense needs to be applied. Performance-enhancing products should not be promoted to children, and parents and coaches bear a responsibility for monitoring and guiding children's behavior in this respect. The Council for Responsible Nutrition (CRN) believes re-sponsible regulation by the Food and Drug Administration (FDA) and by the states is needed to support consumer confidence in dietary supple-ments, including sports nutrition products. FDA has the necessary au-thority, and needs only to exercise it constructively.

Safe performance enhancement

Creatine is probably the best-studied performance-enhancing supple-ment. . . . Creatine has been shown to improve performance measurably, when a quick burst of energy is required, and it is for this reason that it is widely used by collegiate and weekend athletes. While more study can always be done, there is no evidence that creatine use is unsafe in otherwise healthy people. It should not be used by people with kidney problems.

[The] media falsely asserts that dietary supplements, including sports nutrition products, are "unregulated."

Ephedra is an herbal supplement containing naturally-occurring ephedrine alkaloids. It provides an energy boost and has been widely used to provide the extra "oomph" that some people need to pursue a regular exercise program. It also contributes to weight loss, and two recent studies conducted jointly by researchers at Columbia and Harvard demonstrated that ephedra can be used safely and effectively for weight loss, at levels up to 90 milligrams (mg) of ephedra alkaloids per day. A recent comprehensive safety evaluation supported by CRN and conducted by Cantox, one of the leading firms in toxicological analysis. The Cantox study concluded that ephedra is safe at levels such as those used in the Harvard/Columbia study, using a risk assessment method developed by the National Academy of Sciences. The study evaluated all the available safety evidence, including FDA's adverse event reports. CRN has submitted the Cantox study to FDA, to help the agency complete its effort to establish new regulations for ephedra-containing supplements.

The industry supports most of the existing state regulations on ephedra product formulation and labeling. The state regulations require an extensive warning label, cautioning against use by people with risk factors such as hypertension or heart disease, and the industry voluntarily adopted such labeling as early as 1995. The state regulations that impose a dosage limit generally select a maximum of 100 mg per day—a level very similar to that supported by the Harvard/Columbia studies and the Cantox report. If FDA's regulatory proposal had followed this model, the regulation would be in place by now. The basis for the agency's more restrictive approach has been criticized not only by industry but by a General Accounting Office report issued in 1999.* "CRN urges FDA to revise its approach to the regulation of ephedra and move forward promptly to conclude the rulemaking based on sound and unbiased scientific analysis, including the Cantox report," said Dr. John Hathcock, CRN's vice president for nutritional science and regulatory affairs.

Androstenedione is a hormone precursor and therefore may present more potential concerns, simply because there needs to be more research on all its effects. In the studies done so far, its conversion to hormones and the body's own production of those same hormones seem to be controlled by feedback mechanisms which help protect against excess. A comprehensive safety assessment would be helpful.

Consumer Reports, like many other media, falsely asserts that dietary supplements, including sports nutrition products, are "unregulated" and says they are readily available in all kinds of stores because of the Dietary

---

* Editor's note: In 1997, the FDA proposed limiting the amount of ephedrine alkaloids in ephedra products and requiring safety labels that recommended a dosage limit of 24 mg per day. As of spring 2002, no regulations have been put into effect.

Supplement Health and Education Act of 1994 (DSHEA). "In fact, FDA has as much authority over the safety and labeling of dietary supplements as it does over any other food product, and all foods and supplements have been freely sold in all types of stores *forever,* not just since 1994," said Dr. Annette Dickinson, CRN's vice president for scientific and regulatory affairs. She added, "The critics' rants against DSHEA are so sweeping they have become ludicrous. The truth is that dietary supplements are used by more than half of Americans, are beneficial in a variety of ways, and have a safety record comparable to that of any other food category."

16

Genetic Engineering May One Day Replace Performance-Enhancing Drugs

Jere Longman

Jere Longman is a sportswriter for the New York Times.

Sports authorities are concerned that athletes may begin to employ genetic engineering techniques to enhance their athletic performance. Although gene therapy is still at an early stage of development, athletes looking for a competitive edge may not wait for science to perfect safe applications. A single insertion of genetic material could potentially bulk up muscles for years at a time, precluding the need to take continual cycles of performance-enhancing drugs. Testing athletes for altered genes would also be difficult and require invasive detection methods. Gene therapy is adding to the ethical debate over whether athletes should be allowed to alter their fundamental makeup to become more competitive.

For three decades, the International Olympic Committee (I.O.C.) has been engaged in a game of chemical cat-and-mouse. Athletes use drugs to enhance their performances, scientists devise tests to identify those drugs, then the athletes move on to more sophisticated doping techniques.

Now, the rules of the game may be changing, leaving the Olympic committee even further behind.

Gene therapy and athletes

Concerned that athletes would soon employ genetic engineering in attempting to run faster, to jump higher and to throw farther, the I.O.C. and the affiliated World Anti-Doping Agency are about to convene inaugural meetings on the subject. "For once we want to be ahead, not behind," Dr. Patrick Schamasch of France, the I.O.C.'s medical director, said.

Genes serve as a script that directs the body to make proteins. It seems fantastic today to think that injecting a gene could result in more fast-twitch muscle fibers, enabling a sprinter to run 100 meters in six seconds instead of just under 10. Or injecting a gene that could increase oxygen-carrying capacity so that a marathoner could run 26.2 miles in one and a half hours instead of just over two. Some scientists and Olympic committee officials believe genetic engineering in sports is a decade away. Some believe it may appear in two years. Still others believe crude forms might already be in use, at great health risk to athletes.

"I think certain methods could have already started," said Johann Olav Koss, the 1994 Olympic speed skating champion from Norway who is a member of the I.O.C. and a doctor.

Athletes, who are often eager for an edge in competition, are not very likely to wait for science to perfect gene therapy.

Medical applications of gene therapy—efforts to cure or prevent disease—are at a very rudimentary stage, with only one form of gene therapy having been shown conclusively to work. Little is understood about the implications of introducing genes into a human body, so any use aimed at improving athletic performance would now be considered dangerous and unethical.

But the human genome has been mapped out and the technology, however immature, is evolving rapidly. Athletes, who are often eager for an edge in competition, are not very likely to wait for science to perfect gene therapy. Inherently, athletes are risk takers. And there is enormous financial pressure and reward to win, to produce records and to keep up with other athletes who are succeeding through illicit means.

Genetic engineering in sport will foster not only a greater potential health risk for athletes than does conventional doping, but also a greater potential for performance enhancement, said Dr. Jacques Rogge, a Belgian surgeon who is an I.O.C. delegate and vice chairman of its medical commission. Instead of repeatedly ingesting pills or taking injections, an athlete may be able, with a single insertion of genetic material, to sustain bulked-up muscle mass or heightened oxygen-carrying capacity for months or even years. Such genetic manipulation would be extremely difficult, if not virtually impossible, to detect using current methods, scientists said.

Ethical questions abound

At the coming meetings of the Olympic committee and the anti-doping agency, officials will discuss the potential benefits and risks of genetic engineering and the potential detection methods, and they will face a number of ethical questions. Should genetic manipulation be banned entirely in sport? Should it be allowed for athletes healing from injury or recovering from disease? If the technology can be made safe, do healthy athletes have the right to engineer themselves like race cars to push the boundaries of achievement? Will two classes of competition be needed?

"What if you're born with something having been done to you?" Maurice Greene of Los Angeles, the Olympic champion at 100 meters, said. He wondered, would manipulation of an egg or an embryo be considered cheating? "You didn't have anything to do with it," he said.

The Olympic committee scheduled a meeting for June 6, 2001, on genetic engineering only after the anti-doping agency announced plans for its own gathering in September, an apparent political gesture to appear out front on the issue, said Dr. Arne Ljunqvist of Sweden, who is an I.O.C. delegate and chairman of the anti-doping agency's medical, health and research committee.

The second meeting is considered the more significant of the two; the agency hopes to gather three dozen athletes, sports scientists, genetics experts, ethicists and policy officials from the Food and Drug Administration and the National Institutes of Health in Cold Spring Harbor, N.Y.

"For the first time, a substantial group of people involved in sports administration, sports science and genetic science will sit around the same table and discuss a common potential problem," Dr. Ljunqvist said.

The concerns range from the pragmatic to the philosophical. Do the Olympic committee and other sports organizations have the willpower or financial resources to combat the use of genetic engineering? The total cost of conventional drug tests are already about $1,000 each.

The insertion of a gene . . . could theoretically turn the body into [a performance-enhancing drug] factory.

Ultimately, at the heart of the issue will be a profound question: what is a human athlete?

"What are the endpoints of manipulation?" said Dr. Theodore Friedmann, director of the gene therapy program at the University of California at San Diego and a member of the anti-doping agency's health and research committee. "Is the hope to incrementally sneak up on the one-and-a-half-minute mile? Or six seconds for 100 meters? Is the question, How fully can we engineer the human body to do physically impossible things? If it is, what do you have at the end of that? Something that looks like a human, but is so engineered, so tuned, that it's no longer going to do what the body is designed to do."

Anything for an edge?

Athletes, scientists and sports administrators agree that someone will attempt genetic engineering, if they have not already. Concern over health and safety issues has not been a strong deterrent to the epidemic use of conventional performance-enhancing drugs.

In a 1995 survey, nearly 200 aspiring American Olympians were asked if they would take a banned substance that would guarantee victory in every competition for five years and would then cause death; more than half answered yes.

A seminar on teenage steroid use, held in New York City, revealed these desperate efforts to boost athletic performance: A female basketball player asked a doctor to break her arms and reset them in a way that might make them longer; pediatricians were being pressured by parents to give their children human growth hormone to make them taller and perhaps more athletic; doctors were being asked by the parents of football players to provide steroids so their sons might gain college scholarships.

Only a change in cultural attitudes will curb genetic engineering, just as a cultural shift has led to an intolerance for smoking.

A molecular scientist, speaking on condition of anonymity, said in an interview that a foreign exchange student staying with the scientist's family was approached at a swimming pool by a stranger and was told, "You are absolutely beautiful; I'll give you $35,000 for one of your eggs." The student accepted the offer. It is not inconceivable that some parent looking to create an elite athlete would offer far more money for such an arrangement with, say, Marion Jones, the world's fastest woman.

"In theory, you could do in vitro fertilization, stick in a gene for x, y or z and you've built a kid," the scientist said. "It's been done in mice. But I'd consider that brave new world stuff. It's not happening with humans."

Other techniques now being tested on lab animals seem much less futuristic. For instance, the gene that codes for the hormone erythropoietin, or EPO, has been identified. Produced by the kidneys, EPO regulates the production of red blood cells. A synthetic version can serve as a wonder drug for patients suffering from anemia, AIDS or cancer. Because it enhances oxygen-carrying capacity, EPO is believed to be in widespread use in such endurance sports as cycling and distance running.

Conventional illicit doping measures require athletes to be injected at regular intervals with EPO to maintain the endurance benefit. The insertion of a gene, however, could theoretically turn the body into an EPO factory. Last year a study by Dr. Steven M. Rudich, a transplant surgeon then at the University of California at Davis, indicated that a single injection of the EPO gene into the leg muscles of monkeys produced significantly elevated red blood cell levels for 20 to 30 weeks.

"An athlete would be out of his mind to want to use this," Dr. Rudich, who is now at the University of Michigan, said. Ruefully, he said about genetic engineering in sports, "I bet it exists."

Muscular mice

Genetic material can be delivered to the body by several methods. Dr. Rudich took a weakened virus, inserted a snippet of EPO gene, then injected it into the monkeys' thigh muscles. Each gene consists of DNA, the ladder-like structure that serves as a genetic carpenter, instructing the body what to construct. In this case, the DNA signaled the muscles to produce EPO, which stimulated the production of red blood cells.

Other hormones and proteins that can be used in gene therapy for performance enhancement are human growth hormone and a protein called insulin-like growth factor-1, or IGF-1. Growth hormone can be used to treat dwarfism in children and to prevent muscle loss in the aging process. IGF-1 is critical to the repairing of muscle tissue. Both substances are believed to be used illicitly now by athletes using conventional methods to increase muscle size and strength.

Ten years ago, Dr. Helen Blau of Stanford demonstrated that a gene could be introduced into a mouse to stimulate production of normal levels of human growth hormone in the bloodstream for as long as three months, compared with 10 minutes if the drug were taken directly. Recently, she and others showed that oral antibiotics could be used as a switch to turn the gene on and off.

"In theory, it is possible that an athlete could be genetically engineered to have a gene so you could increase muscle strength, train with it and shut it off when you want to, which would make drug testing more difficult," said Dr. Blau, chairwoman of the department of molecular pharmacology at Stanford Medical School. "Whether it's happened, I have no idea. In theory, it's possible. It's something to keep an eye on. It could be a future concern for the Olympics."

A 1998 study by scientists at the University of Pennsylvania and Harvard involving IGF-1 used gene therapy in mice to halt the depletion of muscle and strength that comes with old age. Older mice increased their muscle strength by as much as 27 percent in the experiment, which suggested possibilities for athletes as well as for preserving muscle strength in elderly people and increasing muscle power in those who suffer from muscular dystrophy.

"We called them Schwarzenegger mice," said Dr. Nadia Rosenthal, an associate professor at Harvard Medical School and a co-author of the study. It has since been demonstrated that mice enhanced with the IGF-1 gene continue to gain size and strength when exercising on a wheel without any apparent adverse health effects, she said.

"I'd be totally surprised if it was not going on in sports," Dr. Rosenthal said, speaking generally of crude attempts at genetic engineering. "Those with terminal cancer and AIDS want to know, 'What will keep me alive?' Athletes want to know, 'What will make me win?'"

Hidden dangers

The danger in attempting genetic engineering now for athletics, Dr. Rosenthal and other researchers cautioned, is that experiments with mice and monkeys might not work the same way in humans and might lead to negative side effects.

If a gene for producing EPO cannot be shut off properly, the blood will begin to thicken with excessive red blood cells and that could cause strokes and heart attacks.

If the gene for human growth hormone is not regulated, muscles might grow until they outstripped the blood supply or overwhelmed tendons and ligaments. Misuse could also lead to heart and thyroid disease and cause the size of someone's head, jaw, hands and feet to increase dramatically.

The entire process of genetic engineering remains imprecise. Dr. Thomas Murray, president of the Hastings Center, a biomedical ethics research institute in Garrison, N.Y., likened it to firing at the bull's-eye of a target with a spray of shotgun pellets. It is not known exactly where the virus and DNA go when injected, how they get where they are going or what the body's immune response will be.

An attempt to strengthen the shoulder muscles of a javelin thrower, for instance, might lead inadvertently to an enlargement of the heart muscle. Or worse. A teenager died in 1999 during a therapeutic study at the University of Pennsylvania, apparently in reaction to the virus carrying genes intended to treat a metabolic disorder.

"We don't know the technology well enough even to be sure what's happening in a therapeutic setting," Dr. Friedmann of California-San Diego said. "We certainly don't know the technology well enough to know how safe a gene is going to be to an athlete."

Before athletes are fitted with designer genes, the next advance may be to create more synthetic versions of drugs like EPO and growth hormone that mimic the effects of genetic engineering, scientists said. But genetic manipulation of the human body for sport is sure to come. The question is, to what extent?

Michael Johnson, the Olympic sprinting champion, said he thought the health risks would scare off many athletes. Werner Franke, a German molecular biologist who helped bring to light the systematic doping of athletes by East Germany, said he was not particularly worried about genetic engineering because chemical footprints left by the inserted virus and DNA would facilitate detection.

The most effective argument against genetic enhancement may be that it will coerce others to alter their fundamental makeup . . . if they want to compete.

"I think it will be mostly science fiction," Mr. Franke said. He accused the I.O.C. of "purposely barking up the wrong tree" in an attempt to camouflage its lack of commitment to catching athletes who cheat by conventional methods.

Many scientists, however, disagree with Mr. Franke's assessment of the potential ease of detecting altered genes. With available technology, they say, scientists would have to know exactly where the gene was inserted in order to identify it, which would most likely require muscle biopsies.

"No athlete in his right mind is going to allow himself to be probed here and there for evidence of a virus," Dr. Friedmann said.

Eventually, some noninvasive detection methods might be developed, like chemical markers or a chip that could be encoded with the sequence of a specifically altered gene. But some researchers believe that only a change in cultural attitudes will curb genetic engineering, just as a cultural shift has led to an intolerance for smoking.

"We have to change the fundamental mind-set about doping," Dr.

Don Catlin, who operates the Olympic drug-testing lab at the University of California at Los Angeles, said.

There appears to be little fear that human cloning will have a significant effect in sport. If say, Michael Johnson were cloned, the result would almost certainly not be the same world record-setter as the original, researchers say, because environmental, nutritional and motivational factors also play significant roles in developing athletes.

"If I'm the clone of Michael Johnson, I've got to bend myself into all sorts of shapes to run, because genetically that's what I'm destined to be," Dr. Friedmann said. "I run and run and run, and I can't ever get anywhere. Then what am I? I'm a Michael Johnson who can't run. That's a nobody. That must be a crushing experience to learn you're not what you're genetically destined to be."

Moral and athletic limits

Cloning aside, many athletes and sports officials say they would abhor genetic engineering in sport. "It is supposed to be a test of human capability, not a chemical war or a genetic war," Brandi Chastain of the American women's soccer team said.

If genetic engineering is used, "then sport is dead," said Dr. Bengt Saltin, director of the Center for Muscular Research at Copenhagen University in Denmark.

Yet, American society tolerates other types of enhancement, from the caffeine stimulation of coffee to breast enlargement to erectile function. And although there has been an outcry about genetically engineered corn, there was mass celebration when Mark McGwire broke the major league home run record in 1998 using androstenedione, a steroid precursor that is banned by the Olympics and many professional sports.

"Nobody cared about what McGwire was using," said Jon Drummond, a member of the victorious American 4x100-meter relay team at the Sydney Olympics. "They just wanted to see him break the record."

If genetic engineering can be made safe, with fewer side effects even than conventional methods of doping, it may grow increasingly difficult to find supportable arguments against using gene alteration to achieve excellence in sport, Dr. Friedmann said.

"Our society has already decided partly that maybe there isn't a lot wrong with it, and that we can build ourselves, change ourselves, as much as we'd like, consistent with safety and medical ethics," he said. "If a weight lifter makes massive muscles and with a flinch of the finger can lift a few hundred pounds, what's wrong with that ethically? I'm not sure you'll get good answers to that."

Not all athletes will have equal access to genetic engineering, but not all of them have equal access today to the same nutrition and training facilities. Not every distance runner, for instance, can train at altitude. Should sea-level athletes be allowed to take EPO to match the oxygen-carrying benefits for those who live at altitude?

The most effective argument against genetic enhancement may be that it will coerce others to alter their fundamental makeup, perhaps at great risk, if they want to compete.

"The argument in favor of allowing people to do this is based on our

American tradition of giving individuals a huge amount of autonomy over their own bodies," said Dr. Eric Juengst, an ethicist at Case Western Reserve University in Cleveland. "The limits on that kind of freedom are interpersonal. Once your actions cross the line of affecting just yourself and begin to affect other people, we have license to step in."

That right to set moral limits, however, will inevitably clash with a desire to break athletic limits. Anyone who could run 100 meters in six seconds "has no place in sports," said Mr. Greene, the world record-holder at 9.79 seconds. But, he added, "If anyone can run the 100 in six seconds, I'd like to see it."

Organizations to Contact

The editors have compiled the following list of organizations concerned with the issues debated in this book. The descriptions are derived from materials provided by the organizations. All have publications or information available for interested readers. The list was compiled on the date of publication of the present volume; the information provided here may change. Be aware that many organizations take several weeks or longer to respond to inquiries, so allow as much time as possible.

Athletes Training & Learning to Avoid Steroids (ATLAS)
Division of Health Promotion and Sports Medicine
Oregon Health & Science University
3181 SW Sam Jackson Park Rd., CR110, Portland, OR 97201-3098
(503) 494-8051 • fax: (503) 494-1310
e-mail: hpsm@ohsu.edu • website: www.ohsu.edu

ATLAS is a program designed by researchers at the Oregon Health Sciences University to discourage the use of anabolic steroids and other performance-enhancing drugs by male high school athletes. The program is administered to sports teams through peer instructors and coaches and is implemented through schools, recreational centers, and community organizations. ATLAS has been tested on over 3,200 students and has shown significant results in reducing steroid and supplement use.

Canadian Centre for Ethics in Sport (CCES)
1600 James Naismith Dr., Suite 205, Gloucester, ON K1B 5N4 Canada
(613)748-5755 • fax: (613)748-5746
e-mail: info@cces.ca • website: www.cces.ca

The CCES strives to promote drug-free sports in Canada and in international competitions. It produces and disseminates educational materials on performance-enhancing drugs and administers drug testing in Canadian athletic programs.

International Olympic Committee (IOC)
Chateau de Vidy, CH-1007 Lausanne, Switzerland
fax: 011-41-21-621-6216
website: www.olympic.org

The IOC administers the Olympic Games. Its anti-doping code, updated in January 2000, prohibits the use of performance-enhancing drugs and maintains a list of banned substances. Its website includes information on banned substances, the World Anti-Doping Agency established in November 1999, and other related matters.

National Center for Drug Free Sport
810 Baltimore, Suite 200, Kansas City, MO 64105
(816) 474-8655 • fax: (816) 502-9287
e-mail: Info@drugfreesport.com
website: www.ncaa.org

The National Center for Drug Free Sport administers drug tests required by the National Collegiate Athletic Association. It can provide updated information on banned substances and drug testing procedures.

National Clearinghouse for Alcohol and Drug Information
PO Box 2345, Rockville, MD 20847-2345
(800) 729-6686 • fax: (301) 468-6433
e-mail: shs@health.org • www.health.org

The clearinghouse distributes publications of the U.S. Department of Health and Human Services, the National Institute on Drug Abuse, and other federal agencies. Publications include *Tips for Teens About Steroids* and *Anabolic Steroids: A Threat to Body and Mind.*

National Collegiate Athletic Association (NCAA)
6201 College Blvd., Overland Park, KS 66211-2422
(913) 339-1906
website: www.ncaa.org

The NCAA is the administrative body overseeing intercollegiate athletic programs. It provides drug education and drug testing programs. Information on its bylaws can be found on its website. The NCAA's publications include the *Guide for the College Bound Student-Athlete.*

National Strength and Conditioning Association
1955 N. Union, Colorado Springs, CO 80909
(719) 632-6722 • fax: (719) 632-6367
e-mail: nsca@usa.net • website: www.nsca-lift.org

The association seeks to facilitate an exchange of ideas related to strength development among its professional members. The association offers career certifications, educational texts and videos, as well as the bimonthly journal *Strength and Conditioning*, the quarterly *Journal of Strength and Conditioning Research*, and the bimonthly newsletter *NSCA Bulletin*. Its website includes an index of articles on ergogenic aids, including anabolic steroids.

OATH
1235 Bay St., Fourth Floor, Toronto, ON M5R 3K4 Canada
(877) 843-6284 • fax: (416) 534-7690
e-mail: oath@interlog.com • website: www.theoath.org

OATH is an independent international athlete-led organization that seeks to preserve the ideals of the Olympics, and to provide past and present Olympic athletes a united voice on doping and other issues. It has issued reports on Olympic reforms on anti-doping strategies.

Office of National Drug Control Policy
Executive Office of the President
Drugs and Crime Clearinghouse
PO Box 6000, Rockville, MD 20849-6000
e-mail: ondcp@ncjrs.org • website: www.whitehousedrugpolicy.gov

The Office of National Drug Control Policy is responsible for formulating the government's national drug strategy and the president's antidrug policy. It has worked to improve procedures for preventing drug use in sports. Drug policy studies are available upon request or at its website.

UK Sports Council
40 Bernard St., London, WC1N 1BR United Kingdom
011 020 7841 9500
e-mail: info@uksport.gov.uk • website: www.uksport.gov.uk

The UK Sports Council works to promote and support British athletes in world competitions and to promote anti-doping strategies and ethical standards in sports. Its publications include *Competitors and Officials Guide to Drugs and Sport.* More information is available on its website.

United States Anti-Doping Agency (USADA)
1265 Lake Plaza Dr., Colorado Springs, CO 80906
(866) 601-2632 • fax: (719) 785-2001
e-mail: webmaster@usantidoping.org • website: www.usantidoping.org

The USADA manages the drug testing of U.S. Olympic, Pan Am Games, and Paralympic athletes and enforces sanctions against athletes who violate drug laws. The agency promotes educational programs to inform athletes of the rules governing the use of performance-enhancing drugs, the ethics of doping, and its harmful effects.

United States Olympic Committee (USOC)
One Olympic Plaza, Colorado Springs, CO 80909-5746
fax: (719) 578-4654
website: www.usoc.org

The USOC is a nonprofit private organization charged with coordinating all Olympic-related activity in the United States. It works with the International Olympic Committee and other organizations to discourage the use of drugs in sports. Information on its programs is available on its website.

World Anti-Doping Agency (WADA)
Av. du Tribunal-Federal 34, 1005 Lausanne, Switzerland
(41-21) 351 02 25 • fax: (41-21) 329 15 05
e-mail: info@wada-ama.org • website: www.wada-ama.org

The WADA was created in 1999 as an independent international anti-doping agency. The agency works with international sports federations, national and international Olympic committees, governments, and athletes to coordinate a comprehensive drug testing program. WADA has begun conducting unannounced, out-of-competition tests that it believes will reduce the prevalence of drugs in the Olympics and other international competitions.

Websites

Healthy Competition Campaign
www.healthycompetition.org

The website is part of a public education program launched by the Blue Cross and Blue Shield Association, a federation of health insurers, and provides information on performance-enhancing drugs for teens, parents, and coaches.

International Drugs in Sport Summit
www.dcita.gov.au/drugsinsport

This website includes information and papers presented at a November 1999 summit of government officials hosted by the Australian Minister for Sport and Tourism.

SteroidAbuse.org
www.steroidabuse.org

A service of the National Institute on Drug Abuse (NIDA), this website provides information and articles on the health risks of taking anabolic steroids.

Steroidlaw.com
www.steroidlaw.com

Steroidlaw.com provides health and legal information to those curious about using steroids. Its director, criminal attorney and former bodybuilder Rick Collins, advocates the reform of current steroid laws and contends that the health risks of steroids have been exaggerated.

Bibliography

Books

Charlie Francis	*Speed Trap: A Track Coach's Explosive Account of How the World's Greatest Athletes Win*. New York: St. Martin's, 1990.
Bob Goldman	*Death in the Locker Room II*. Chicago: Elite Sports Medicine Publications, 1992.
John M. Hoberman	*Mortal Engines: The Science of Performance and the Dehumanization of Sport*. New York: The Free Press, 1992.
Barry Houlihan	*Dying to Win: Doping in Sport and the Development of the Anti-Doping Policy*. Strasbourg, France: Council of Europe Publishing, 1999.
Cynthia Kuhn, Scott Swartzwelder, and Wilkie Wilson	*Pumped: Straight Facts for Athletes About Drugs, Supplements and Training*. New York: W.W. Norton & Company, 2000.
Lee F. Monaghan	*Bodybuilding, Drugs and Risk*. New York: Routledge, 2001.
Judy Monroe	*Steroid Drug Dangers*. Berkeley Heights, NJ: Enslow Publishers, 2000.
Elizabeth Ann Nelson	*Coping with Drugs and Sports*. New York: Rosen Publishing Group, 1999.
Rodney G. Peck	*Drugs & Sports*. Center City, MN: Hazelden Informational & Educational Services, 1998.
Steven Ungerleider	*Faust's Gold: Inside the East German Doping Machine*. New York: St. Martin's Press, 2001.
Robert O. Voy with Kirk D. Deeter	*Drugs, Sport, and Politics*. Champaign, IL: Human Kinetics Publishers, 1990.
Ivan Waddington	*Sport, Health, and Drugs*. New York: Routledge, 2000.
Melvin H. Williams	*The Ergogenics Edge: Pushing the Limits of Sports Performance*. Champaign, IL: Human Kinetics Publishers, 1997.
Charles E. Yesalis	*Performance-Enhancing Substances in Sport and Exercise*. Champaign, IL: Human Kinetics Publishers, 2002.
Charles E. Yesalis and Virginia S. Cowart	*The Steroids Game*. Champaign, IL: Human Kinetics Publishers, 1998.

Periodicals

Alan Abrahamson	"Olympics: Former Head of Anti-Doping Campaign Says Nothing Has Changed Since the '80s," *Los Angeles Times*, June 17, 2000.

Sharon Begley and Martha Brant	"The Real Scandal," *Newsweek*, February 15, 1999.
Karen Birchard	"Why Doctors Should Worry About Doping in Sport," *Lancet*, July 4, 1998.
Kim Clark and Robert Milliken	"Positive on Testing," *U.S. News & World Report*, August 14, 2000.
Helen Elliott	"Olympic Scene; Once Again, Drugs Move the Spotlight Off Sports," *Los Angeles Times*, March 4, 2001.
Rob Fernas	"NCAA Testing for New Target; Drugs: Supplements Such as Ephedrine Have Become Biggest Problem for Colleges, Which Use Random Procedures," *Los Angeles Times*, August 16, 2001.
Mike Freeman	"N.F.L. Is Seeing Fewer Flaws in Testing Players for Drugs," *New York Times*, October 7, 2001.
Karen Goldberg Goff	"Despite Sensitive Testing, Athletes Still Dope to Win," *Insight on the News*, March 15, 1999.
Steve Hummer	"Stain of Drugs Persists Sydney 2000: Summer Olympics Special Section," *Atlanta Journal-Constitution*, September 25, 2000.
Armen Keteyian	"Mass Deception," *Sport*, August 1998.
Steve Kettmann	"Berlin Dispatch: Girlz II Men," *New Republic*, July 3, 2000.
Kathiann M. Kowalski	"Steer Clear of Steroid Abuse," *Current Health*, March 1999.
Robert Lipsyte	"Bodybuilding Insider's Straight Talk on Drugs," *New York Times*, May 13, 2001.
Frank Litsky	"Criticism Is Leveled at U.S. Drug Testing," *New York Times*, February 5, 2002.
Jere Longman	"Drug Testing in U.S. Comes Under Fire from Olympic Officials," *New York Times*, September 27, 2000.
Jere Longman	"The Guilty and the Not-So-Innocent," *New York Times*, July 29, 2001.
Maclean's	"The Tour De Shame: The Sports World Reels from New Drug Scandals," August 10, 1998.
Stephanie Mencimer	"Scorin' with Orrin," *Washington Monthly*, September 2001.
William Nack	"The Muscle Murders," *Sports Illustrated*, May 18, 1998.
C.W. Nevius	"Not Your Uncle's Protein Shakes," *San Francisco Chronicle*, July 7, 2001.
Mike Penner	"Olympics: Critics at Drug Summit Also Call for Proposed Anti-Doping Agency to Operate Independently of Committee," *Los Angeles Times*, February 3, 1999.

Andrew Phillips	"The Olympic Drug Cloud: Were These the Shame Games—or the Start of a Real Crackdown on Doping?" *Maclean's*, October 9, 2000.
Rick Reilly	"The 'Roid to Ruin," *Sports Illustrated*, August 21, 2000.
Ray Sahelian	"Androstenedione: Home Run or Hype?" *Better Nutrition*, October 1999.
Richard Sandomir	"I.O.C. Finds Banned Substances in Many Food Supplements," *New York Times*, October 12, 2001.
Joannie M. Schrof	"McGwire Hits the Pills: Brawn-Building Supplements Also Deliver Serious Risks," *U.S. News & World Report*, September 7, 1998.
Seattle Times	"Get Tough on Olympic Drug Tests for NBA, NHL," March 8, 2001.
Amy Shipley	"Anti-Doping Fight May Be Long Battle; International Agency, New Tests Are Coming," *Washington Post*, September 23, 1999.
Gary Smith	"Gotta Catch 'Em All: Armed with New Methods for Detecting EPO, Graham Trout and His Colleagues at Australia's Sports Drug Testing Lab Have Olympic Cheaters in Their Crosshairs," *Sports Illustrated*, September 18, 2000.
Mark B. Stephens	"Ergogenic Aids: Powders, Pills, and Potions to Enhance Performance," *American Family Physician*, March 1, 2001.
E.M. Swift	"Drug Pedaling," *Sports Illustrated*, July 5, 1999.
Time	"Are Drugs Winning the Games?" September 11, 2000.

Internet Articles

Matt McGrath and Gaetan Portal	"New Drugs Give Cheats the Edge," *BBC News*, January 30, 2000. http://news.bbc.co.uk
Stephen A. Shoop and Mike Falcon	"Steroids: Teens Feeling Pressure to Bulk Up," *USA Today*, December 27, 1999. www.usatoday.com

Index

Adolescent Training and Learning to Avoid Steroids (ATLAS), 44
adrenocorticotrophic hormone (ACTH), 16
  testing for, 18
aggression
  as side effect of steroids, 43–44, 72–74
Alzado, Lyle, 36
amphetamines, 17, 30
anabolic-androgenic steroids
  abuse of, by teens is a growing problem, 41–44
  classes of, 43
  examples of, 13
  psychological dependence and, 74
  research on, is unreliable, 66–67
  side effects of, 13–14, 42
    in teens, 68
    in women, 67
    see also health risks, of steroids
androgens
  excess, adverse effects of, 68–70
  see also anabolic-androgenic steroids
androstenedione, 88, 89, 92
Armstrong, Lance, 52
artificial oxygen carriers, 16
Ashford, Evelyn, 52
athletes
  are tarnished by performance-enhancing drugs, 28–34
  nonsteroid using, should be banned, 60–61
  surveys of, on attitudes toward doping, 36–37, 96–97
  will never stop using performance-enhancing drugs, 20–23
Aubier, Nicolas, 10

Bahrke, M.S., 73
Bailey, Donovan, 27
Bannister, Roger, 58, 59
Barnard, Matt, 20
Baxter, Alain, 8
beta-2 adrenergic agonists
  types and side effects of, 14
Blau, Helen, 98
blood doping, 16
blood testing, 81
Bobet, Louison, 62
Brochard, Laurent, 31
Brown-Séquard, Edouard, 30

Buffet, Marie-George, 32

Catlin, Don, 56, 100
Chastain, Brandi, 100
Coe, Seb, 24, 26
Collins, Rick, 65
Consumer Reports (magazine), 92
corticosteroids, 16, 53
cortisone, 16
Coubertin, Pierre de, 29
Council for Responsible Nutrition, 91
Cowart, Virginia, 66, 72, 73
creatine, 91–92
crime
  link with steroid use, 73–74

Darling, Devaughn, 89
Death in the Locker Room: Steroids & Sports (Goldman), 66
Declaration on Principles of Health Care for Sport Medicine (World Medical Association), 47
Delignieres, Bruno, 47
Dianobol, 8
Dickenson, Annette, 93
Dietary Supplement Health and Education Act of 1994, 92–93
dietary supplements
  lack of regulation of, 89–90
  performance-enhancing
    are dangerous, 88–90
    are safe, 91–93
DiPasquale, M.G., 75
diuretics
  avoiding drug detection with, 86
doping
  as challenge to public health/medicine, 33
  definition of, 28
  history of, 29–30
  solutions to problem of, 26–27
Downey, Eamon, 24
Drugs, Sport, and Politics (Voy), 8, 84
Drummond, Jon, 100
Duchaine, Dan, 68

East Germany
  sport doping in, 41–42, 50–53, 54, 58
Economist (magazine), 35
Engquist, Ludmila, 76
ephedra, 92

epitestosterone, 17–18
erythropoietin (EPO), 15, 30
  difficulty in testing for, 56–58
  genetic engineering and, 98
  testing for, 19
ethics
  of genetic engineering, 95–96
  medical, performance-enhancing drugs
    compromise, 45–49
European Commission, 28
Exum, Wade, 42

Faber, Francois, 62
Faust's Gold (Ungerleider), 50
Festina affair, 30–32, 46, 63
Fife, Graeme, 62
Food and Drug Administration, 89
Francis, Charlie, 52, 54
Franke, Werner, 99
Freudenrich, Craig, 11
Friedmann, Theodore, 96, 99, 100

gas chromatography, 18, 87
Gendin, Sidney, 60
genetic engineering
  dangers of, 98–100
  may replace performance-enhancing
    drugs, 94–101
  moral and athletic limits of, 100–101
Geneva Declaration (World Medical
  Association), 48
Gimeno, Andrea, 30
Gimondi, Felice, 31
Gladwell, Malcolm, 50
Goldberg, Karen, 10
Goldman, Bob, 36, 37, 66
Greene, Maurice, 96, 101
El Guerrouj, Hicham, 58, 59

Hathcock, John, 92
health risks
  of beta-2 adrenergic agonists, 14
  of steroids, 13–14
    aggressive/psychiatric symptoms,
      72–74
    have been exaggerated, 65–75
    on heart, 71–72
    on liver, 70–71
    on prostate, 72
heart
  anabolic steroid effects on, 71–72
heroin, 29–30
Hicks, Thomas, 30
Hoberman, John, 9
Höppner, Manfred, 54
human chorionic gonadotropin (hCG),
  14
human genome, 95
human growth hormone (hGH), 15, 30

difficulty in testing for, 55
genetic engineering and, 98
testing for, 18
Hunter, C.J., 8

immuno-assays, 18–19
insulin, 15
insulin-like growth factor (IGF-1), 15
  genetic engineering and, 98
International Olympic Committee
  (IOC), 94
  antidoping conference of, 32
  substances banned by, 7

Jensen, Knut Enemark, 30
Johnson, Ben, 9, 26, 27, 30, 35, 52, 54
Johnson, Michael, 99
Jones, Marion, 97
Joyner, Florence Griffith, 26, 55
Juengst, Eric, 101
Junren, Ma, 38

Kerr, Robert, 53
Kettridge, Richard, 22
Kimmage, Paul, 10
Knacke-Sommer, Christiane, 9, 50, 51
Knapp, Gwen, 88
Koch, Marita, 52
Koss, Johann Olav, 95

Lapize, Octave, 62, 63
Laquer, Ernest, 30
Lewis, Carl, 26, 35
libido
  steroid effects on, 68–69
Lindon, Arthur, 30
Liotard, Philippe, 45
liver
  anabolic steroid effects on, 70–71
Ljunqvist, Arne, 96
Longman, Jere, 94
luteinizing hormone (LH), 14–15
  testing for, 18

Madden, Terry, 77, 78
Masback, Craig, 26
mass- and strength-building drugs,
  13–15
Massi, Rodolfo, 31
mass spectrometry, 18, 87
McCaffrey, Barry, 78
McGwire, Mark, 20–21, 23, 88, 100
McNutt, R.A., 71
media
  influence on sports, 33
Medibolics (magazine), 70
medical ethics
  performance-enhancing drugs
    compromise, 45–49

Melandrini, Giovanna, 32
Merckx, Eddy, 62
Merode, Alexandre de, 37
Mitchell, Dennis, 25
morphine, 30
Mortal Engines: The Science of Performance and Dehumanization of Sport (Hoberman), 9
Morton, Oliver, 62
Murray, Thomas H., 46, 99

narcotics, 16
National Institute on Drug Abuse, 42
Noden, Merrell, 24
Nuremberg Rules, 45

Oakes, Judy, 37
Oldfield, Brian, 53
Olympic Games
    Atlanta (1996), 27, 36, 55
        drug testing at, 23
    drug abuse is rampant in, 77
    history of doping in, 29–30
    need for zero-tolerance policy by, 76–78
    Seoul (1988), 26, 35, 52
    Sydney (2000), 57
Otto, Kristin, 58
Ovett, Steve, 24
oxygen-increasing drugs, 15–16

pain-masking drugs, 16
Pantani, Marco, 31
performance-enhancing drugs
    athletes are tarnished by, 28–34
    athletes will never stop using, 20–23
        con, 24–27
    ban on, should continue, 35–40, 76–78
        con, 50–59, 60–61
    classes of, 12
    compromise medical ethics, 45–49
    drugs masking, 17–18
    genetic engineering may replace, 94–101
    parallel Olympics for athletes using, 62–64
    reasons athletes use, 12–13
    solutions to problem of, 26–27
        random testing, 78
    sports associated with, 36
        weightlifting, 83–85
    testing methods for, 18–19
Picotte, Michael, 78
Pierce, Nicholas, 21, 22
plasma expanders, 18
Powell, John, 26
Price, Robert, 75
prostate

anabolic steroid effects on, 72
protein hormones
    to increase oxygen in tissues, 15
    for masking pain, 16

Raducan, Andrea, 8, 78
relaxants, 17
Reynolds, Butch, 25, 38, 54–55
Rosenthal, Nadia, 98
Rossel, Bruno, 31
Rough Ride: Behind the Wheel with a Pro Cyclist (Kimmage), 10
Rudich, Steven M., 97
Ryckaert, Eric, 31

Saltin, Bengt, 100
Samaranch, Juan Antonio, 23
Schamasch, Patrick, 95
secretion inhibitors, 18
Simpson, Tommy, 21, 30
Smith, Michelle, 25, 40
somatomedin-C. *See* insulin-like growth factor
Speed Trap (Francis), 52, 54
sponsors
    attitudes of, toward doing drugs, 39–40
    encourage drug taking, 23
Sport, Health, and Drugs (Waddington), 8
Sports Illustrated (magazine), 36
Starr, Mark, 76
steroids
    athletes who don't use, should be banned, 60–61
    costs of, 61
    dangers of, are minimal, 60–61
    vs. honest effort, 59
    side effects of, 42
    see also anabolic-androgenic steroids
Steroids Game, The (Yesalis and Cowart), 66
stimulants, 16, 17
Strock, Greg, 9
surveys
    of athletes, on attitudes toward doping, 36–37, 96–97
    on teen use of steroids, 42–43
swimming
    prevalence of doping in, 36

Taylor, Angella, 52, 53
teenagers
    steroid abuse by
        adverse effects of, 68
        is a growing problem, 41–44
Tellez, Tom, 26
Terrados, Nicholas, 31
testing
    avoiding detection by, 56, 82, 85–86

is ineffective, 79–87
methods for, 18–19
overview of, 80–81
problems with, 54–55
random, as key to prevention, 78
testosterone, 13, 30, 47
    difficulty in testing for, 55–56, 84–85, 86
    excess, adverse effects of, 69–70
    see also anabolic-androgenic steroids
Tour de France, 7, 10, 21, 25, 62
    Festina affair and, 30–32, 46, 63
Tour de France (Fife), 62
track and field
    prevalence of doping in, 36

Ungerleider, Steven, 41, 50, 52
urine samples
    contamination of, 54
    obtaining, 81–82
U.S. Anti-Doping Agency (USADA), 11

Verroken, Michelle, 23, 37
Virenque, Richard, 31

Voet, Willy, 7, 31, 63
Voy, Robert, 8, 84

Waddington, Ivan, 8
websites
    on steroid abuse, 44
weight control drugs, 17
weightlifting
    drug use and, 83–85
Wheeler, Rashidi, 89, 90
Whetton, John, 21
women
    use of anabolic steroids by, 67
World Anti-Doping Agency (WADA), 7, 94
    establishment of, 32
World Health Organization, 48
World Medical Association, 46–47, 48
Wright, J.E., 73

Yesalis, Charles, 53, 66, 72, 73, 89, 90

Ziegler, John B., 8
Zulle, Alex, 31